MW01206496

Healthy Eating For Kids

By Don Orwell

http://SuperfoodsToday.com

Your Free Gift

As a way of saying thanks for your purchase, I'm offering you my FREE eBook that is exclusive to my book and blog readers.

Superfoods Cookbook - Book Two has over 70 Superfoods recipes and complements Superfoods Cookbook Book One and it contains Superfoods Salads, Superfoods Smoothies and Superfoods Deserts with ultra-healthy non-refined ingredients. All ingredients are 100% Superfoods.

It also contains Superfoods Reference book which is organized by Superfoods (more than 60 of them, with the list of their benefits), Superfoods spices, all vitamins, minerals and antioxidants. Superfoods Reference Book lists Superfoods that can help with 12 diseases and 9 types of cancer.

http://www.SuperfoodsToday.com/FREE

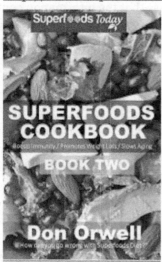

Table of Contents

Introduction

Hello,

My name is Don Orwell and my blog SuperfoodsToday.com is dedicated to Superfoods lifestyle. I had some life changing experiences in 2009 and that led me to start rethinking my eating habits and my current lifestyle. Our son was diagnosed with ADHD around that time too. He was born end of 2002 and in September 2008 he started primary school. After a few months we got a call from his teacher and she explained that he is not focused in school and has all symptoms of ADHD (Attention deficit hyperactivity disorder). A few months of consultations confirmed that he has ADHD. My wife started to search for anything that can help alleviate symptoms, hoping that we can avoid Ritalin and other medications. Nutrition search discovered that some foods can fuel ADHD. Also, our friends found out at the same time that their 3-year-old son is autistic and they already started to take nutritional measures to alleviate autism and that included gluten free and casein free diet. They said that he is noticeably better behaving since being on that diet (lower hyperactivity, less temper tantrums, he started to make eye contact and his speech improved) and we decided to learn everything we could about foods that fuel ADHD.

When I started my research, I kept hitting info about high sugar intake, blood sugar levels, insulin sensitivity, cholesterol levels, fast food diet that most Americans are used to, processed foods, ingredients in processed food and so on. It turned out that the same food that was causing my problems was the food that is fueling ADHD. Sugar, processed food and refined carbs. Then I compiled the list of whole foods that is healthy and can help with my problems and my son's ADHD. When I started to research each food more closely, I kept hitting web sites that dealt with superfoods. When the list was completed, I found out that all the food from my list were superfoods. This is how Superfoods diet was born.

Eating habits are learned behaviors. What your children learn to eat at home early in life stays with them forever. Kids under 2 years of age easier accept new foods, so start as early as possible. Most research says that it takes an average of <u>ten to twelve attempts</u> before a child will try a new food.

Problem with todays' western diet is that we are disconnected from whole food sources and we rely on processed food too much. <u>67% of calories in the Western diet come from wheat, corn and soy!!</u> Compare that to the diet 100 or 200 years ago!! Fewer and fewer people cook meals from scratch because it's easier and faster to throw a frozen dinner in the oven or get something from a fast-food restaurant on the way home from work. That is an easy way. But we have to strive to provide a variety, moderation, and balance to your kids menu. We have to be good role models. In order to be good role model we must <u>educate ourselves</u> first and then practice what we preach. Take kids with you when you go grocery shopping. Let them decide which fruit they will eat. While we always want to make the healthiest choices for our children's bodies, a special treat (ice cream) once a week won't do any damage.

Kids don't need French fries, Doritos and pizza to keep them happy. Highly processed foods like these are loaded with chemicals, synthetic fats, additives, artificial sweeteners, and food colorings. Food colorings and additives are fueling ADHD. Unfortunately, you can't keep heavily processed foods out of their diets forever. <u>But</u> the longer you limit exposure while teaching those healthy eating habits, the more likely your children will be to make better choices when left to their own. Don't use food as rewards, bribes, or punishments, stickers work just as well.

Let kids help in the kitchen. Offer them a variety, cut veggies in ribbons, julienne them or cut in any weird shapes you can think of. Let them dip veggies in hummus or pesto or salsa or guacamole, those condiments are all healthy compared to ketchup full of corn syrup or mayonnaise full of soy oil. Also, timing is important, if they're hungry, they're less picky. Enforce a 3 bites rule. I was able to get my kids try anything and if they didn't like it, they were allowed to stop after 3 bites. If everything else fails, sneak healthy ingredients.

My kids eat some veggies only when they are cut differently than usual. They will eat carrots cut like spaghetti, but not plain carrots. I discovered by chance that they liked carrot spaghetti mixed within salad with green leafy spinach and lettuce. But they didn't want to eat a salad, they tried to fish out the carrot spaghetti out of a salad and eat only them. Next day I served only carrot spaghetti on a plate thinking that they'll be delighted, but they didn't want to eat them. They said that carrot spaghetti doesn't taste the same as yesterday. What the heck? Then I figured out, they were covered with salt and olive oil, so I added some salt and olive oil. Nope, they're not fun to eat, they want to fish them out of the big bowl of green leaves. So, we let them do that. They ate tons of carrot that evening. On any other day they would eat leafy green salad without complaining, but on the next few days all they wanted was to fish out the carrot spaghetti out of a salad. Luckily, after some time they started to eat a mixture of spinach and carrot spaghetti and they eat it ever since. With broccoli we had a different story. They didn't want broccoli in their soup. Carrot is fine, but not the broccoli. I mean, soup cooked with broccoli tastes different, but they will eat it, they just don't want to see the broccoli in their soup bowls. But if I serve them cooked broccoli without soup, drizzled with olive oil and a little bit of salt, they will eat it. Somehow olive oil and a little bit of salt over any veggie, cooked or uncooked, does wonders with my kids.

Next example. My daughter likes to eat nuts as a snack and oatmeal with milk for breakfast. But she won't eat them mixed all in one hot breakfast, if the nuts and flax seed are ground. Her explanation is that the ground nuts are scratching her throat. Go figure. So, we serve nuts as a snack, flax meal goes in some other dishes and we don't enforce them for breakfast. I personally love to eat hot milk & oatmeal breakfast with 1 tbsp of grounded nuts, seeds, flax meal and some cinnamon and cocoa.

What olive oil and salt are for veggies, raw honey is for fruits. Pour a little bit of raw honey on the fruit they don't like and they will eat it.

My daughter is generally pickier than my son. She won't eat fruits that are not ripe or ones that are passed their prime. So, we serve her fruits that are in season. Cutting fruits and veggies in different shapes helped when they were small and they're eating now pretty much any veggie or fruit. The point is: don't stop trying, serve kid's fruits and veggies in all possible shapes and occasions and eventually they will accept it. My daughter eats raw cooking onions for breakfast!?! I would never think that she might do something like that, but she keeps asking and we give it to her. But only if they're cut in wedges, so go figure. She'll eat them in any form in salad, but if they're served separately, she wants them in wedges. Although her teacher complained a few times that she had bad breath in the morning, she keeps eating it with savory dishes for breakfast. Her favorite salad is one medium sized onion cut in small pieces, 1 tomato or 1 cup any green leafy vegies, covered with Superfoods yogurt dressing mixed with 100 grams of soft farmers' cheese. I mix the yogurt dressing and the cheese first and form a thick paste (consistency of a mayo, she actually calls this mix a healthy mayo and it does tastes like mayo if you put slightly more olive oil) and then I fold the veggies and mix until they're properly covered. That salad is a complete meal for her, she is not asking for anything else with it.

And last but not least, sneak a lot of Omega-3 rich food into their meals; it boost brain power. I'm adding flax meal to anything I make and surprisingly, it doesn't scratch their throat when sneaked in cooked rice or stew.

A few words about ADHD. Before switching to superfoods, we noticed how much food additives and artificial colors affected our son. During and after kids' birthdays, where he would gobble Doritos, Coke and Spiderman colored birthday cakes, he would become virtually impossible to handle. He wouldn't listen to anyone and he'd be the hyperactive poster child. We tried virtually everything, gluten free diet, casein free diet, both of them at the same time and noticed that gluten free diet improved his behavior immediately. We reintroduced superfoods dairy product (low-fat Greek yogurt, kefir and low-fat farmers' cheese) into his diet and noticed that he was still behaving great. But the most important change was when we excluded all processed food from our diet and started to eat only whole food superfoods. That was the period when we abandoned Play Attention and self-concluded that he doesn't have ADHD anymore. Of course, we were wrong, but his behavior now is almost perfect. He still makes noises, sometimes louder that we'd prefer, but that is the only ADHD related behavior that we can spot. His school behavior is great, he's focused, motivated and people who don't know him from his ADHD period don't suspect that he was diagnosed with ADHD. If your child has ADHD and you're already on casein free diet, you can exclude dairy ingredients from superfoods recipes and replace them with other ingredients. For example, you can replace yogurt in any of the recipes with light tahini sauce (tahini, olive oil, lemon juice, salt, eventually diluted with little water if necessary). For stronger tahini sauce add ground cumin, minced garlic and chopped cilantro. Farmers or cottage cheese can be replaced with hummus, guacamole or red pepper dip.

When I decided to write this book, I excluded all recipes that both of my kids don't like (curries, roasted beets salad, Brussels sprout recipes and similar). E.g. my daughter doesn't like mushrooms except on pizza, but I included mushrooms recipes because my son will eat no matter how they are prepared. Same thing with shrimps and some other ingredients, one of my kids likes it, the other does not. But there is a chance that you will some recipes that your kids will eat. Perennial favorites for both of my kids are anything made with minced meat (meatloaf, meatballs, grilled beef patty with salad etc.), anything that includes plain yogurt, most of stir fries, all of "grilled meat & salad" meals, anything "breaded", anything patty shaped (crab cakes), oatmeal and eggs breakfasts, desserts and anything with brown rice.

Switch to Superfoods!

Well, this is it, you don't have any processed food in your house, you're stocked on fresh veggies, fruits and other healthy stuff and you're ready to change your life! Congratulations for willingness to get healthier and better looking you!! Please remember these common facts:

Breakfast Veggies: When I'm referring to breakfast veggies, I mean some red or yellow pepper stripes, cucumber and pickles. If you want, you can eat celery, green onions (spring onions) and sauerkraut, I eat them with eggs or farmers or cottage cheese. Hey, you can even eat broccoli, cauliflower, lettuce and spinach for breakfast. If you want, you can roast or grill some veggies (eggplant, zucchini and peppers) and have them with savory breakfasts.

Cinnamon: Cinnamon lowers blood sugar, helps maintain insulin sensitivity and is a very powerful antioxidant. Add it every time you eat oatmeal.

Cocoa: Cocoa consumption is associated with decreased blood pressure, improved blood vessel health, and improvement in cholesterol levels. Some people eat dark chocolate; I add it to oatmeal or drink it. Buy unsweetened cocoa, ideally unprocessed one, because processing at high temperature destroy healthy ingredients in it.

Nuts and Seeds: Flax should be always ground. Buy flax meal or grind them with a coffee grinder. Almond is healthiest nut, but you can sometimes eat walnuts, Brazil nuts or pecan instead. It's clever to eat every time a different type of nuts, but remember that almonds are the healthiest ones.

Grilling and Frying: Fry on a little bit of coconut oil in the skillet, 7 to 10 minutes for most of the meat and fish. Don't overdo it. Don't grill for too long. If you don't like the meat suggested in the recipe, replace it with something similar. Use beef instead of pork or chicken instead of fish. Think about organ meats, liver or kidneys, they have more vitamins then meat. If you don't want red meat, use chicken. If you crave fried food, dip the meat in beaten eggs mixture, cover it with flax meal instead of breadcrumbs and bake it in the oven, it's delicious!!

Coconut oil: Use coconut oil. Period. Avoid blended vegetable oils, corn oil and soybean oil. I'm cooking with coconut oil and eat one spoon of coconut oil once a day because of my low thyroid; to me, it tastes like heaven, way better than the Bounty. Coconut oil also fights cancer, it contains MCTs—medium chain triglycerides, who are fighting plaque in the brain. Plaque in the brain is causing Alzheimer's disease. Coconut oil also boost metabolism and it's great for the skin. Some people experience stomach discomfort when taking a spoon of coconut oil on empty stomach, some even vomit. If you experience this, eat coconut oil after meal or mix it in a meal.

Extra-virgin olive oil: Olive oil is the healthiest oil you can buy, as it contains the highest monounsaturated content. Extra-virgin is the oil that results from the first cold pressing of the olives. Being the purest olive oil, it's also the most expensive. But because it has a low smoke point, it should not be used for cooking.

Yogurt and low-fat cheese: Low fat or non-fat Greek (or plain) yogurt is the only one recommended. If you can't find Greek Yogurt, use any plain yogurt. 0.5% or 1% fat Yogurt tastes the best, if you ask me. If you want fruit yogurt, add some fresh berries (or frozen) or fruits in the plain or Greek yogurt and add some Stevia or raw honey if you have to. Doing that, you'll know what exactly went into that snack and you'll avoid industrial chemicals found in fruit yogurts. Choose low-fat farmers cheese over cottage cheese. When choosing Cheddar, Colby or Mozzarella, choose low-fat.

Breads: You would be better off if you avoid any breads, paleo or non-gluten. If you crave something bread like, try egg based flatbreads recipes, like egg pancakes, egg muffins or egg pizza crust or Almond/Tapioca flour naan.

Salad Dressings: Store bought salad dressing contain high fructose corn syrup and soybean oil or canola oil. Forget them. **Forever**. Superfoods dressing would be similar to "Italian Dressing" - olive oil/lemon/minced garlic/salt + some herbs. We'll call second dressing a "Yogurt Dressing" – half a cup of plain low-fat Yogurt or low-fat buttermilk with olive oil/minced garlic/salt. Amount of olive oil I'm using is usually 1 teaspoon per person and the rest is added to taste.

Occasionally I would add a teaspoon of mustard or some herbs like basil, oregano, marjoram, chives, thyme, parsley, dill or mint. If you like spicy hot food, add some cayenne in the dressing. It will speed up your metabolism.

Stir Fry Stir fry meat and veggies in coconut oil. Add some garlic, ginger and half of the onion cut in wedges and season only with fish sauce. If you have to, thicken the sauce with tapioca flour or arrowroot flour.

Condiments Forget about Mayo or Tartar sauce (it's processed food containing refined soybean oil), Ketchup (contains high fructose corn syrup) or BBQ sauce (more high fructose corn syrup then ketchup). Healthy condiments are hummus, salsa, hot sauce, guacamole, mustard and pesto. Use them sparingly in Phase 1.

Broths: Cook broths and freeze. I cook every few weeks a large pot of chicken soup and freeze half of it, because I don't want to eat processed food.

Oatmeal: Buy regular oatmeal, unenriched and not sweetened.

Exotic Superfoods: When people hear that I'm eating only Superfoods they usually comment "Oh, Superfoods are so expensive" thinking on various Superfoods in powder form (Spirulina, Chlorella) or Superfoods berries and seeds (Goji, Chia). When I explain that I eat regular everyday Superfoods such as kale and avocado, they keep asking have I experimented with exotic Superfoods. Yes I have, but I didn't wanted to create recipes where such Superfoods are prominently featured or put them in regular recipes because people will complain that recipe ingredients are expensive. So, I'll list here how I use various exotic Superfoods:

• I add seaweeds to any soup or stew I make and you can do the same with Chlorella and Spirulina. They also can be added to smoothies, condiments and salads. Some people use them in granola recipes or energy bars along with Maca powder.

• I eat Goji berries as a snack or sprinkle them on oatmeal breakfasts and smoothies.

• Wherever flax seeds are used, you can use Chia seeds instead (oatmeal breakfasts, smoothies)

Healthy Eating For Kids

Allergy labels: SF – Soy Free, GF – Gluten Free, DF – Dairy Free, EF – Egg Free, V - Vegan, NF – Nut Free

Condiments

Basil Pesto

- 1 cup basil
- 1/3 cup cashews
- 2 garlic cloves, chopped
- 1/2 cup olive oil

Process basil, cashews and garlic until smooth. Add oil in a slow stream. Process to combine. Transfer to a bowl. Season with salt and pepper. Stir to combine. Allergies: SF, GF, DF, EF, V

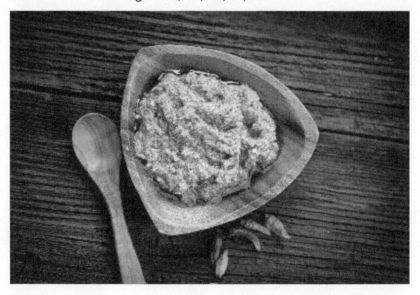

Cilantro Pesto

- 1 cup cilantro
- 1/3 cup cashews
- 2 garlic cloves, chopped
- 1/2 cup olive oil or avocado oil

Process cilantro, cashews and garlic. Add oil in a slow stream. Process to combine. Transfer to a bowl. Season with salt and pepper. Stir to combine. Allergies: SF, GF, DF, EF, V

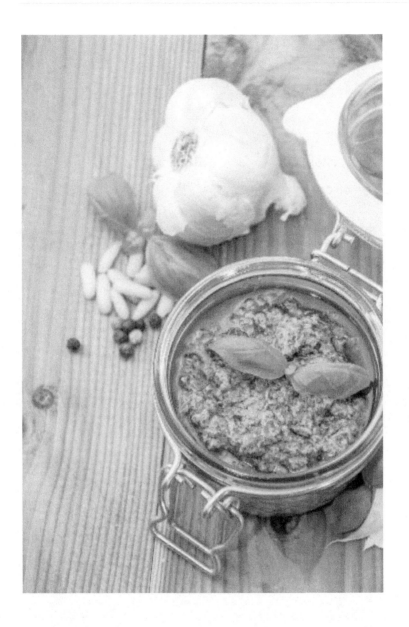

Sundried Tomato Pesto

- 3/4 cup sundried tomatoes
- 1/3 cup cashews
- 2 garlic cloves, chopped
- 1/2 cup olive oil or avocado oil

Process tomato, cashews and garlic. Add oil in a slow stream. Process to combine. Transfer to a bowl. Season with salt and pepper. Stir to combine. Allergies: SF, GF, DF, EF, V

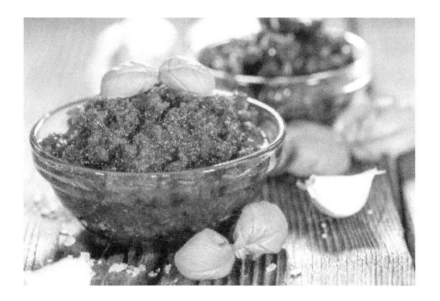

Broths

Some recipes require a cup or more of various broths, vegetable, beef or chicken broth. I usually cook the whole pot and freeze it.

Vegetable broth

Servings: 6 cups

Ingredients

- 1 tbsp. coconut oil
- 1 large onion
- 2 stalks celery, including some leaves
- 2 large carrots
- 1 bunch green onions, chopped
- 8 cloves garlic, minced
- 8 sprigs fresh parsley
- 6 sprigs fresh thyme
- 2 bay leaves
- 1 tsp. salt
- 2 quarts water

Instructions - Allergies: SF, GF, DF, EF, V, NF

Chop veggies into small chunks. Heat oil in a soup pot and add onion, scallions, celery, carrots, garlic, parsley, thyme, and bay leaves. Cook over high heat for 5 to 7 minutes, stirring occasionally.

Bring to a boil and add salt. Lower heat and simmer, uncovered, for 30 minutes. Strain. Other ingredients to consider: broccoli stalk, celery root

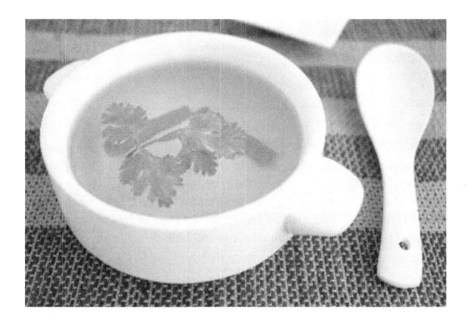

Chicken Broth

Ingredients

- 4 lbs. fresh chicken (wings, necks, backs, legs, bones)
- 2 peeled onions or 1 cup chopped leeks
- 2 celery stalks
- 1 carrot
- 2 sprigs fresh thyme
- 2 sprigs fresh parsley
- 1 tsp. salt

Instructions - Allergies: SF, GF, DF, EF, NF

Put cold water in a stock pot and add chicken. Bring just to a boil. Skim any foam from the surface. Add other ingredients, return just to a boil, and reduce heat to a slow simmer. Simmer for 2 hours. Let cool to warm room temperature and strain. Keep chilled and use or freeze broth within a few days. Before using, defrost and boil.

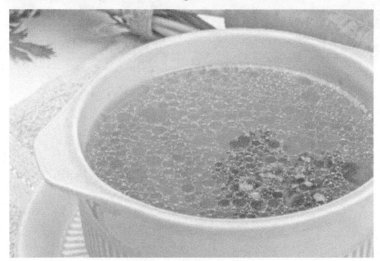

Beef Broth

Ingredients

- 4-5 pounds beef bones and few veal bones
- 1 pound of stew meat (chuck or flank steak) cut into 2-inch chunks
- olive oil or avocado oil
- 1-2 medium onions, peeled and quartered
- 1-2 large carrots, cut into 1-2 inch segments
- 1 celery rib, cut into 1 inch segments
- 2-3 cloves of garlic, unpeeled
- Handful of parsley, stems and leaves
- 1-2 bay leaves
- 10 peppercorns

Instructions - Allergies: SF, GF, DF, EF, NF

Heat oven to 375°F. Rub olive oil over the stew meat pieces, carrots, and onions. Place stew meat or beef scraps, stock bones, carrots and onions in a large roasting pan. Roast in oven for about 45 minutes, turning everything half-way through the cooking.

Place everything from the oven in a large stock pot. Pour some boiling water in the oven pan and scrape up all of the browned bits and pour all in the stock pot.

Add parsley, celery, garlic, bay leaves, and peppercorns to the pot. Fill the pot with cold water, to 1 inch over the top of the bones. Bring the stock pot to a regular simmer and then reduce the heat to low, so it just barely simmers. Cover the pot loosely and let simmer low and slow for 3-4 hours.

Scoop away the fat and any scum that rises to the surface once in a while.

After cooking, remove the bones and vegetables from the pot. Strain the broth. Let cool to room temperature and then put in the refrigerator.

The fat will solidify once the broth has chilled. Discard the fat (or reuse it) and pour the broth into a jar and freeze it.

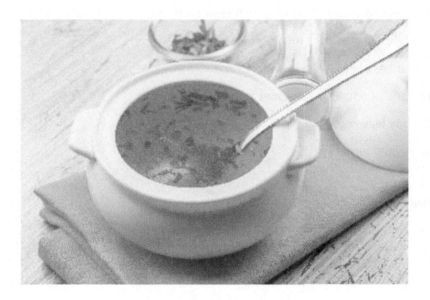

Tomato paste

Some recipes (chili) require tomato paste. I usually prepare 20 or so liters at once (when tomato is in season, which is usually September) and freeze it.

Ingredients

- 5 lbs. chopped plum tomatoes
- 1/4 cup extra-virgin olive oil or avocado oil plus 2 tbsp.
- salt, to taste

Instructions - Allergies: SF, GF, DF, EF, V, NF

Heat 1/4 cup of the oil in a skillet over medium heat. Add tomatoes. Season with salt. Bring to a boil. Cook, stirring, until very soft, about 8 minutes.

Pass the tomatoes through the finest plate of a food mill. Push as much of the pulp through the sieve as possible and leave the seeds behind.

Bring it to boil, lower it and then boil uncovered, so the liquid will thicken (approx. 30-40 minutes). That will give you homemade tomato juice. You get tomato paste if you boil for 60 minutes, it gets thick like store bought ketchup.

Store sealed in an airtight container in the refrigerator for up to one month, or freeze, for up to 6 months.

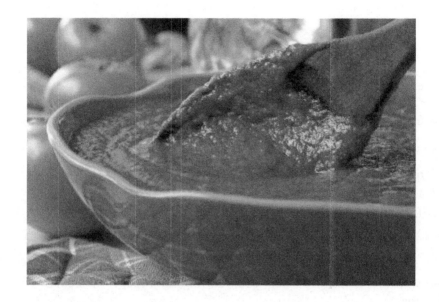

Precooked beans

Again, some recipes require that you cook some beans (butter beans, red kidney, garbanzo) in advance. Cooking beans takes around 3 hours and it can be done in advance or every few weeks and the rest get frozen. Soak beans for 24 hours before cooking them. After the first boil, throw the water, add new water and continue cooking. Some beans or lentils can be sprouted for few days before cooking and that helps people with stomach problems.

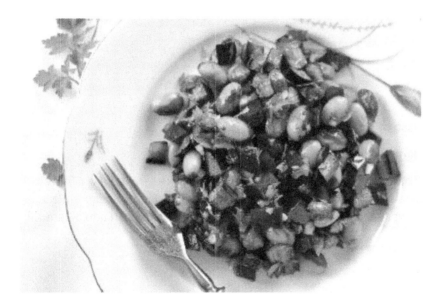

Breakfast - Oatmeal

Oatmeal Breakfasts

Allergy labels: SF – Soy Free, GF – Gluten Free, DF – Dairy Free, EF – Egg Free, V - Vegan, NF – Nut Free

Superfoods Oatmeal Breakfast

Serves 1 - Allergies: SF, GF, DF, EF, V, NF

- 1 cup cooked oatmeal

- 1 tsp. of ground flax seeds

- 1 tsp. of sunflower seeds

- A dash of cinnamon

- Half of the tsp. of cocoa

Cook oatmeal with hot water and after that mix all ingredients. Sweeten if you have to with few drops of raw honey. Optional: You can replace sunflower seeds with pumpkin seed or chia seed. You can add a handful of blueberries or any berries instead of cocoa.

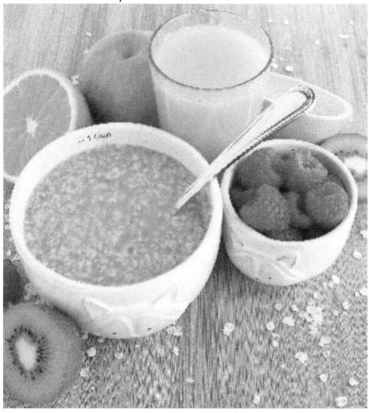

Oatmeal Yogurt Breakfast

Serves 1 - Allergies: SF, GF, EF, NF

- 1/2 cup dry oatmeal

- Handful of blueberries (optional)

- 1 cup of low-fat yogurt

Mix all ingredients and wait 20 minutes or leave overnight in the fridge if using steel cut oats.

Nutrition Facts

Serving Size 247 g

Amount Per Serving

Calories 255	Calories from Fat 37
	% Daily Value*
Total Fat 4.2g	6%
Saturated Fat 2.1g	11%
Cholesterol 11mg	4%
Sodium 131mg	5%
Potassium 557mg	16%
Total Carbohydrates 36.6g	12%
Dietary Fiber 3.6g	15%
Sugars 16.8g	
Protein 14.3g	

Vitamin A 2%	•	Vitamin C 12%
Calcium 35%	•	Iron 10%

Nutrition Grade A

* Based on a 2000 calorie diet

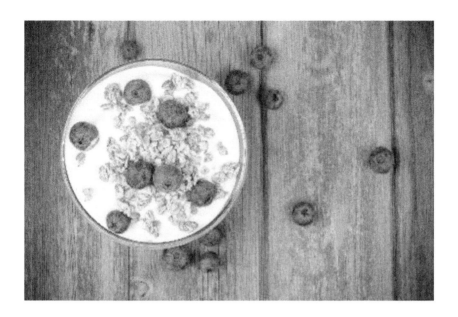

Cocoa Oatmeal

Serves 1

Ingredients - Allergies: SF, GF, DF, NF

- 1/2 cup oats
- 2 cups water
- A pinch tsp. salt
- 1/2 tsp. ground vanilla bean
- 2 tbsp. cocoa powder
- 1 tbsp. raw honey
- 2 tbsp. ground flax seeds meal
- a dash of cinnamon
- 2 egg whites

Instructions

In a saucepan over high heat, place the oats and salt. Cover with 3 cups water. Bring to a boil and cook for 3-5 minutes, stirring occasionally. Keep adding 1/2 cup water if necessary as the mixture thickens.

In a separate bowl, whisk 4 tbsp. water into the 4 tbsp. cocoa powder to form a smooth sauce. Add the vanilla to the pan and stir.

Turn the heat down to low. Add the egg whites and whisk immediately. Add the flax meal, and cinnamon. Stir to combine. Remove from heat, add raw honey and serve immediately.

Topping suggestions: sliced strawberries, blueberries or few almonds.

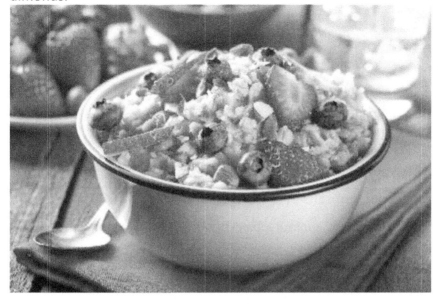

Flax and Blueberry Vanilla Overnight Oats

Serves 1

Ingredients - Allergies: SF, GF, EF, V, NF

- 1/2 cup oats
- 1/4 cup water
- 1/4 cup low-fat yogurt
- 1/2 tsp. ground vanilla bean
- 1 tbsp. flax seeds meal
- A pinch of salt
- Blueberries, walnuts, blackberries, raw honey for topping

Instructions

Add the ingredients (except for toppings) to the bowl in the evening. Refrigerate overnight.

In the morning, stir up the mixture. It should be thick. Add the toppings of your choice.

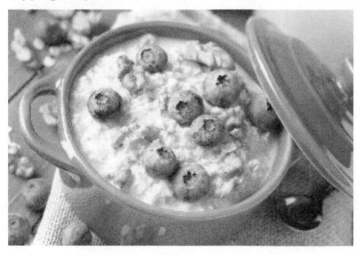

Apple Oatmeal

Serves 1

Ingredients - Allergies: SF, GF, DF, EF, V, NF

- 1 grated apple
- 1/2 cup oats
- 1 cup water
- Dash of cinnamon
- 2 tsp. raw honey

Instructions

Cook the oats with the water for 3-5 minutes.

Add grated apple and cinnamon. Stir in the raw honey.

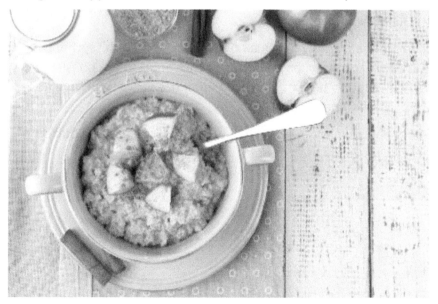

Almond Butter Banana Oats

Serves 1

Ingredients - Allergies: SF, GF

- 1/2 cup oats
- 3/4 cup water
- 1 egg white
- 1 banana
- 1 tbs. flax seeds meal
- 1 tsp raw honey
- pinch cinnamon
- 1/2 tbs. almond butter

Instructions

Combine oats and water in a bowl. Beat the egg white, then whisk it in with the uncooked oats. Boil on stovetop. Check consistency and continue to heat as necessary until the oats are fluffy and thick. Mash banana and add to oats. Heat for 1 minute

Stir in flax, raw honey, and cinnamon. Top with almond butter!

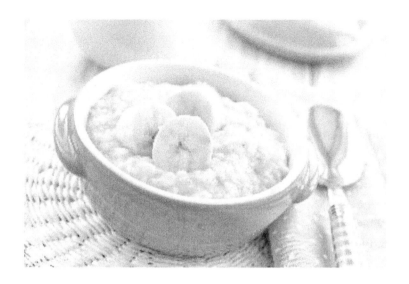

Coconut Pomegranate Oatmeal

Serves 1

Ingredients - Allergies: SF, GF, DF, EF, V, NF

- 1/2 cup oats
- 1/3 cup coconut milk
- 1 cup water
- 2 tbs. shredded unsweetened coconut
- 1-2 tbs. flax seeds meal
- 1 tbs. raw honey
- 3 tbs. pomegranate seeds

Instructions

Cook oats with the coconut milk, water, and salt.

Stir in the coconut, raw honey and flaxseed meal. Sprinkle with extra coconut and pomegranate seeds.

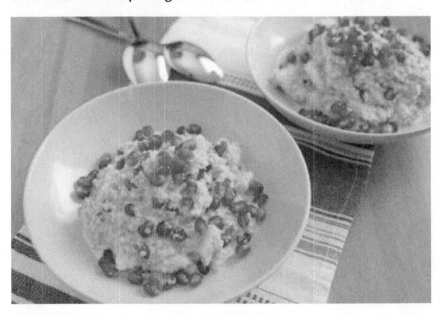

Banana Almond Overnight Oats

Serves 1

Ingredients - Allergies: SF, GF, DF, EF, V

- 1/2 cup oats
- 1/2 cup coconut milk
- 1 banana
- 1 tbs. flax seeds meal
- 1 tsp raw honey
- pinch cinnamon
- 1 tsp dried cranberries, 2 Brazil nuts
- 1/2 tbs. almond butter

Instructions

Make a smoothie with banana, coconut milk, almond butter, honey and cinnamon. Stir in flax and oatmeal and leave overnight. Top with 1 tsp. dried cranberries Brazil nuts.

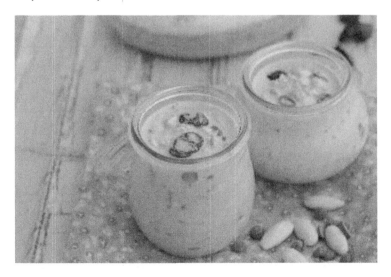

Walnut Oatmeal with Fresh Blueberries

Serves 1

Ingredients - Allergies: SF, GF, DF, EF, V

- 1/2 cup blueberries
- 1/2 cup oats
- 1 cup water
- 1/2 cup walnuts
- Dash of cinnamon
- 2 tsp. raw <u>honey</u>

Instructions

Cook the oats with the water for 3-5 minutes.

Add walnuts and cinnamon. Stir in the raw honey. Top with blueberries

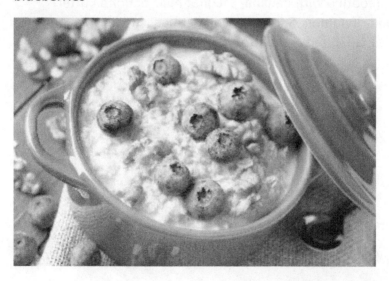

Raspberry Oatmeal

Serves 1

Ingredients - Allergies: SF, GF, DF, EF, V

- 1/2 cup raspberries
- 1/2 cup oats
- 1 cup water
- 1/2 cup sesame seeds
- Dash of cinnamon
- 2 tsp. raw honey

Instructions

Cook the oats with the water for 3-5 minutes.

Add sesame seeds and cinnamon. Stir in the raw honey. Top with raspberries

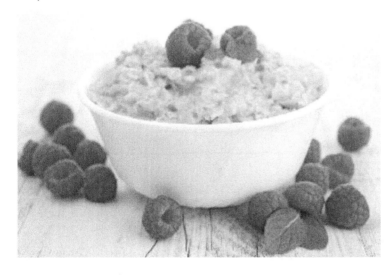

Strawberry Oatmeal

Serves 1

Ingredients - Allergies: SF, GF, DF, EF, V

- 1/2 cup strawberries
- 1/2 cup oats
- 1 cup water
- 2 Tbsp. sunflower seeds
- 1 Tbsp. raisins
- 2 tsp. raw honey

Instructions

Cook the oats with the water for 3-5 minutes.

Add sesame seeds and cinnamon. Stir in the raw honey. Top with raspberries

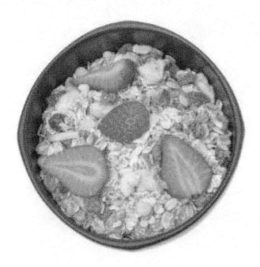

Kiwi Oatmeal

Serves 1

Ingredients - Allergies: SF, GF, DF, EF, V

- 1 sliced kiwi
- 1/2 cup oats
- 1 cup water
- 2 Tbsp. pumpkin seeds
- 1 Tbsp. raisins
- 2 tsp. raw honey

Instructions

Cook the oats with the water for 3-5 minutes.

Add sesame seeds and cinnamon. Stir in the raw honey. Top with raspberries

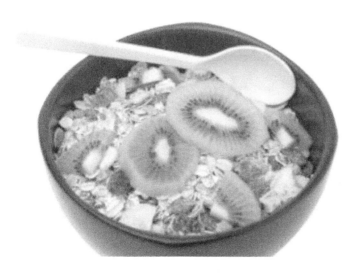

Baked Oatmeal – Cranberry & Walnut

Serves 1

Ingredients - Allergies: SF, GF, EF, V

- 1/2 cup oats
- 1/4 cup water
- 1/4 cup low-fat almond milk
- 1/2 tsp. ground <u>vanilla</u> bean
- 2 tbsp. walnuts
- 1 tsp. coconut oil
- 2 tbsp. dried cranberries

Instructions

Oil small baking dish. Preheat oven to 375F. Mix all the ingredients and pour them to the baking dish. Bake approximately 40 minutes.

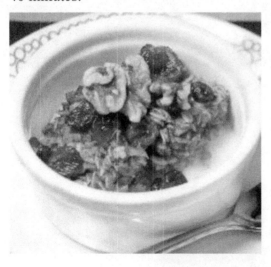

Blueberry Sunflower Seeds Oats

Serves 1

Ingredients - Allergies: SF, GF, EF, V, NF

- 1/2 cup oats
- 3/4 cup water
- 1/4 cup blueberries
- 1/2 tsp. ground vanilla bean
- 2 tbsp. sunflower seeds
- 1 tbsp. raw honey

Instructions

Cook the oats with the water for 3-5 minutes. Mix in vanilla and honey. Top with blueberries and sunflower seeds.

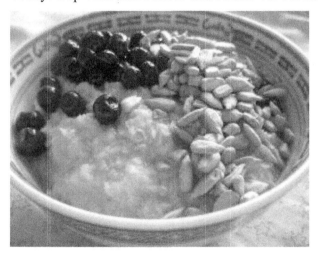

Almonds, Cinnamon & Almond Milk Oatmeal

Serves 1

Ingredients - Allergies: SF, GF, EF, V, NF

- 1/2 cup oats
- 3/4 cup water
- 1/4 cup low-fat almond milk
- 1/2 tsp. cinnamon
- 2 tbsp. whole almonds

Instructions

Cook the oats with the water for 3-5 minutes. Mix in vanilla and honey. Top with blueberries and sunflower seeds.

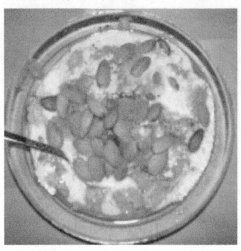

Apple and Cranberry Oatmeal

Serves 1

Ingredients - Allergies: SF, GF, EF, V, NF

- 1/2 cup oats
- 3/4 cup water
- 1/4 cup dried cranberries
- 1/2 tsp. cinnamon
- 1 apple, chopped

Instructions

Cook the oats with the water for 3-5 minutes. Mix in cinnamon, cranberries and apple.

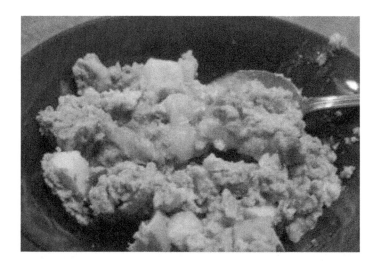

Blue Milk Oatmeal

Serves 1

Ingredients - Allergies: SF, GF, EF, V, NF

- 1/2 cup oats
- 3/4 cup almond milk
- 1/4 cup fresh chopped cranberries
- ½ cup blueberries
- 1 banana, chopped

Instructions

Cook the oats with the almond milk for 3-5 minutes and add blueberries. Mix in cranberries and banana. After some time, blueberries will turn milk blue ☺.

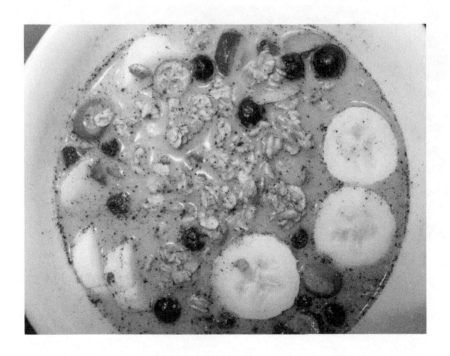

Yogurt, Sesame Seeds and Blueberry Oatmeal

Serves 1

Ingredients - Allergies: SF, GF, EF, V, NF

- 1/2 cup oats
- 3/4 cup yogurt
- 1/4 cup sesame seeds
- 1/2 tsp. cinnamon
- 4 almonds
- 1/2 cup blueberies, chopped

Instructions

Mix yogurt, sesame seeds and oats and let them soak for 15 minutes. Add cinnamon, almonds and blueberries.

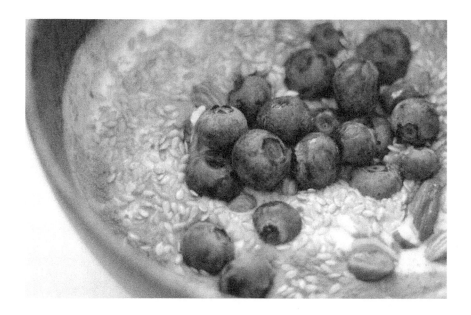

Yogurt, Banana and Almond Oatmeal
Serves 1

Ingredients - Allergies: SF, GF, EF, V, NF

- 1/2 cup oats
- 3/4 cup Yogurt
- 1/4 cup dried blueberries
- 1 Tbsp. sesame seeds
- 6 almonds
- 1 banana, sliced

Instructions

Cook the oats with the water for 3-5 minutes. Mix in cinnamon, blueberries and banana and top with sesame seeds and almond.

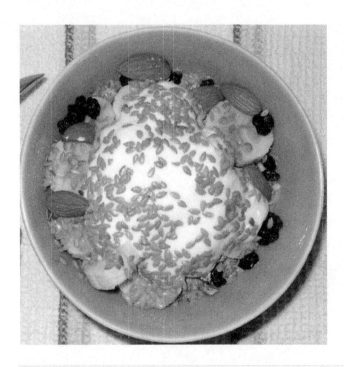

Sweet Baked Breakfasts

Vegan Banana Carrot Bread

Ingredients

- 2 cups almond flour
- 1/3 cup lucuma powder
- 2 teaspoons cinnamon
- 2 teaspoons baking powder
- 1/2 teaspoon baking soda
- Pinch of sea salt
- 2 Tbsp. hemp hearts
- 1/2 cup almond milk at the room temperature
- 1/4 cup warmed coconut oil
- 3 mashed bananas
- 3 carrots, grated
- 3/4 cup chopped walnuts

Instructions

Preheat oven to 350 degrees F. In a large mixing bowl, add flour, honey, cinnamon, baking powder, soda and salt and mix well. Add almond milk, coconut oil, hemp hearts, mashed bananas and mix. Add carrots. Put the mixture in the slow cooker and cook on high for 2 hours or 4 hours on low.

Let cool for 10 minutes, remove from pan and let cool completely. Store covered. Serve warmed or at room temperature. Slices would pair nicely with this Cashew Sweet Cream.

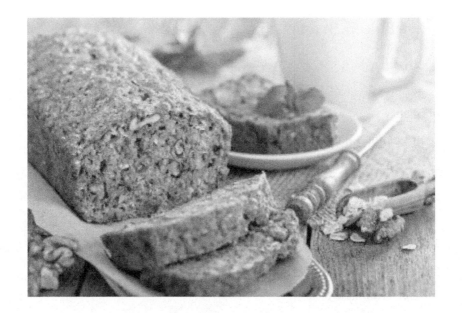

Upside down Apple Cake

Ingredients

Bottom Fruit Layer:

- 2 tbsp. coconut oil, melted
- 1 apple, sliced, or 1/4 cup blueberries, plums, banana etc.
- 2 tbsp. walnut chunks
- 2 tbsp. coconut sugar
- 1 tsp ground cinnamon.

Top Cake Layer:

- 1/3 cup lucuma powder
- 1/4 cup unsweetened coconut milk, or unsweetened almond milk.
- 1 tsp ground vanilla bean
- 1 tsp lemon juice.
- 1 banana, mashed, or 1/4 cup blueberries
- 1/3 cup coconut flour

Instructions

Place 2 tbsps. coconut oil into slow cooker pan. Sprinkle 2 tbsps. coconut sugar all over the oil. Sprinkle 1 tsp cinnamon on top of sweetened layer.

Layer apple slices or blueberries on top of sweetened layer. Add walnut pieces to fruit layer. Set aside.

Combine all the "top cake layer" ingredients in a large mixing bowl except for the coconut flour. Mix and add the coconut flour and mix well.

Spoon batter on top of fruit layer and spread evenly.

Cook on low for 4 hours.

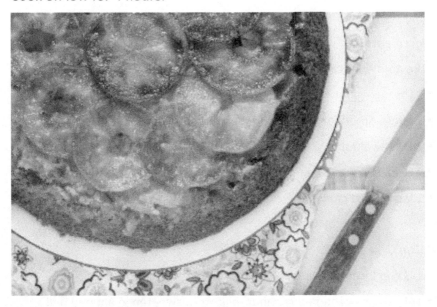

Cheese, Eggs & Raspberry Casserole

Serves 4-6

Ingredients - Allergies: SF, GF, NF

- 1 cup low fat farmers cheese
- 1 cup low fat cream cheese
- 1 cup lucuma powder
- 1 cup low fat sour cream
- 2 large eggs + 3 egg whites
- 2 tablespoons almond flour
- 1 tsp. ground vanilla bean
- 1 cup raspberries
- 1/2 cup black currants or blueberries

Instructions

Preheat the oven to 350 F. Beat both cheeses, lucuma powder and sour cream until smooth (few minutes). Whisk egg whites in a bowl and then add to the cheese mixture along with 2 whole eggs, almond flour, ground vanilla bean and lemon zest. Beat on medium speed for 3 minutes and pour in the oiled casserole dish.

Put strawberries and black currants on top and bake until the cake is set (approx. 60-70 minutes). Turn off the oven and keep the cheesecake inside for 15 minutes.

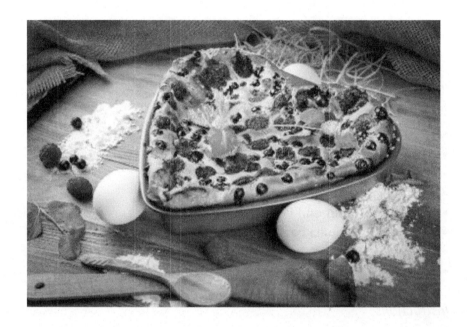

Oatmeal, Walnuts and Cranberry Casserole

Serves 6

Ingredients - Allergies: SF, GF, DF, EF, NF

- 2 cups oats
- 1/2 cup lucuma powder
- 1 tsp. cinnamon
- 1 tsp. baking powder
- 1/2 tsp. salt
- 1 cup walnuts
- 1 egg
- 1/2 cup blueberries
- 1/2 cup raspberries
- 2 cups coconut or almond milk
- 3 Tbsp. coconut oil
- 1 Tbsp. ground vanilla bean

Instructions

Preheat oven to 375 and oil the casserole dish.

Mix oats, lucuma powder, cinnamon, baking powder, salt, walnuts and berries. Whisk together the milk, egg, coconut oil and vanilla in another bowl. Put the oat mixture to the casserole dish and pour milk mixture.

Bake approx. 40 minutes.

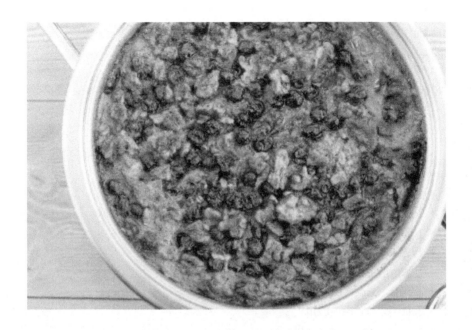

Chia Pudding Recipes

Coconut Chia Pudding

Ingredients

- 1/4 cup Chia seeds
- 1 cup coconut milk
- 1/2 tablespoon Royall jelly
- 1 tsp. Ground Vanilla Bean
- a pinch of Nutmeg
- Top with Blueberries

Instructions

Mix all ingredients except blueberries and leave overnight in the fridge. Top with blueberries.

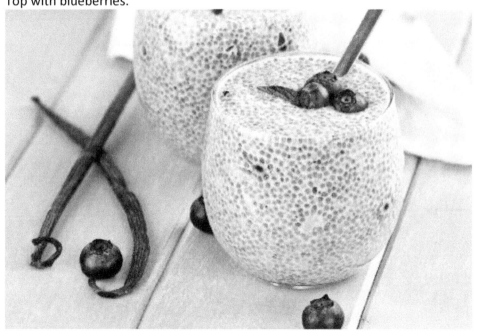

Coconut Pomegranate Chia Pudding

Ingredients

- 1/4 cup Chia seeds
- 1 cup Coconut milk
- 1/2 tablespoon Raw honey
- 1/2 tablespoon Coconut flakes
- Top with Pomegranate seeds

Instructions

Mix all ingredients except pomegranate and leave overnight in the fridge. Top with pomegranate.

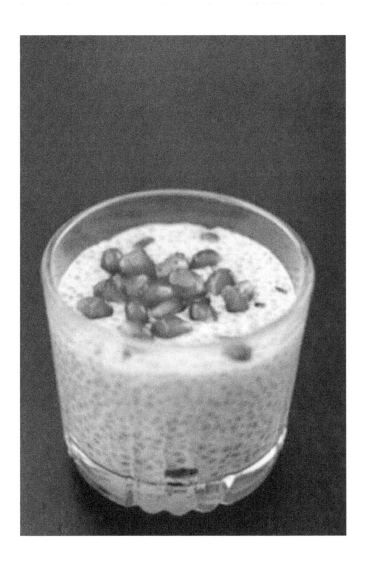

Yogurt & Mango Chia Pudding

Serves 2

Ingredients

- 1/4 cup Chia seeds
- 1 1/2 cup yogurt
- 1 tablespoon Raw honey
- 1/2 cup chopped Mango

Instructions

Mix 1 cup of yogurt, honey and chia seeds and leave overnight in the fridge. Divide into 2 glasses, top each with 1/4 cup yogurt and 1/4 cup mango.

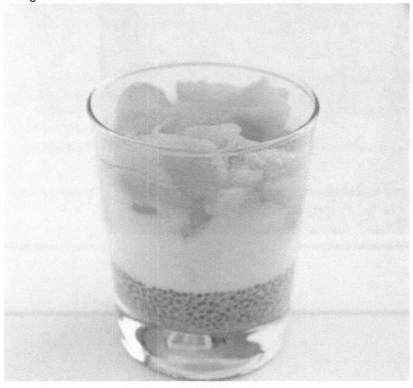

Cacao & Raspberry Chia Pudding

Serves 2

Ingredients

- 1/4 cup Chia seeds
- 1 cup coconut milk
- 1 tablespoon Raw honey
- 1 Tsp. cacao powder
- 1/2 cup yogurt
- 1/2 cup raspberries

Instructions

Mix coconut milk, honey, cacao and chia seeds and leave overnight in the fridge. Divide into 2 glasses, top each with 1/4 cup yogurt and 1/4 cup raspberries.

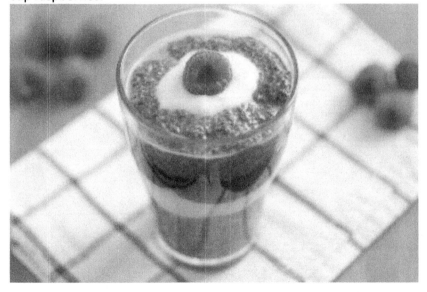

Blueberry Chia Pudding

Serves 2

Ingredients

- 1/4 cup Chia seeds
- 1 cup coconut milk
- 1 tablespoon Raw honey
- 1/2 cup blueberry smoothie
- 1/4 cup chopped almonds

Instructions

Mix coconut milk, honey, blueberry smoothie and chia seeds and leave overnight in the fridge. Divide into 2 glasses and top each almonds.

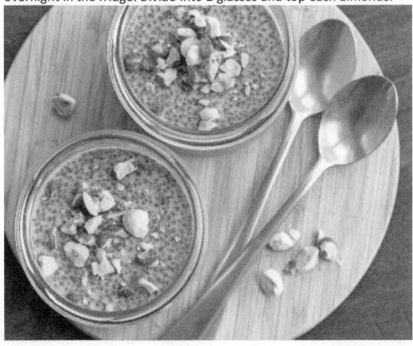

Almond Milk & Cinnamon Chia Pudding

Serves 2

Ingredients

- 1/4 cup Chia seeds
- 2 cups unsweetened almond milk
- 1 tablespoon Raw honey
- 1 tsp. cinnamon
- 1/4 cup slivered toasted almonds and few berries for topping

Instructions

Mix almond milk, honey, cinnamon & chia seeds and leave overnight in the fridge. Divide into 2 glasses and top each with almonds and berries.

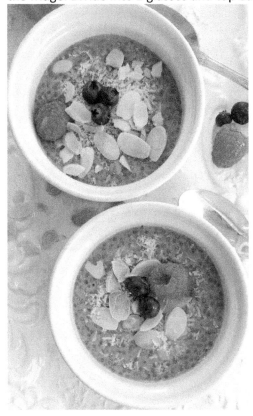

Mixed Berries Chia Pudding

Serves 2

Ingredients

- 1/4 cup Chia seeds
- 2 cups coconut milk
- 1 tablespoon Raw honey
- 1/2 cup mixed berries
- 1/4 cup chopped walnuts

Instructions

Mix coconut milk, honey and chia seeds and leave overnight in the fridge. Divide into 2 glasses and top each with berries and walnuts.

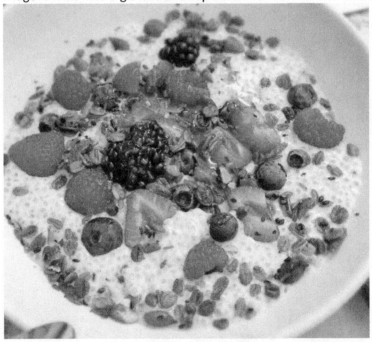

Yogurt Blueberry Chia Pudding

Serves 2

Ingredients

- 1/4 cup Chia seeds
- 2 cups yogurt
- 1/2 cup blueberries & 1 strawberry
- 1/4 cup sunflower, pumpkin and sesame seeds

Instructions

Mix yogurt and chia seeds and leave overnight in the fridge. Divide into 2 glasses and top each berries and seeds.

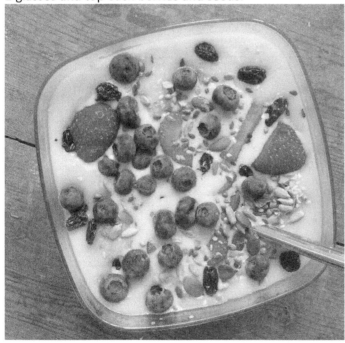

Savory Breakfasts

Serves 1

Regular egg recipes

Allergies: SF, GF, DF, NF

Eggs are great way to start a day and you can enjoy them hard boiled, scrambled, poached or in the omelet with veggies. Eat some breakfast veggies with eggs.

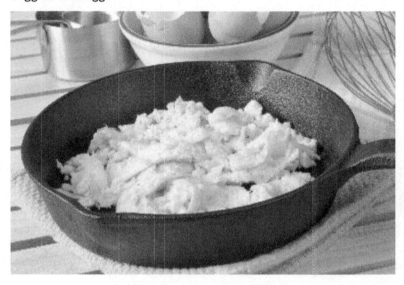

Omelet with Leeks

Serves 1 - Allergies: SF, GF, DF, NF

Cook leeks in little coconut oil until they get soft and then mix the beaten eggs in.

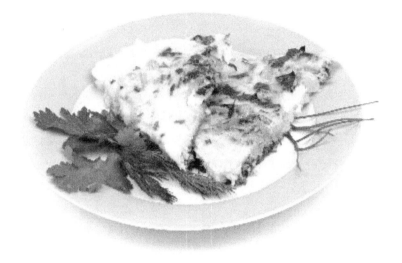

Egg pizza crust

Ingredients - Allergies: SF, GF, DF, NF

- 3 eggs
- 1/2 cup of coconut flour
- 1 cup of coconut milk
- 1 crushed garlic clove

Mix and make an omelet.

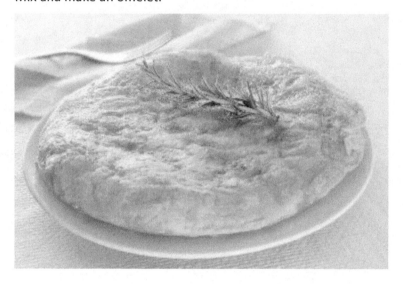

Omelet with Superfoods veggies

Serves 1

Ingredients - Allergies: SF, GF, DF, NF

- 2 large eggs

- Salt

- Ground black pepper

- 1 tsp. olive oil or avocado oil

- 1 cup spinach, cherry tomatoes and 1 spoon of yogurt cheese

- Crushed red pepper flakes and a pinch of dill (optional)

Instructions

Whisk 2 large eggs in a small bowl. Season with salt and ground black pepper and set aside. Heat 1 tsp. olive oil in a medium skillet over medium heat. Add baby spinach, tomatoes and cook, tossing, until wilted (Approx. 1 minute). Set aside. Add eggs and cook until set. Add veggies and cheese on top of eggs. Flip eggs over cheese and veggies. Sprinkle with crushed red pepper flakes and dill.

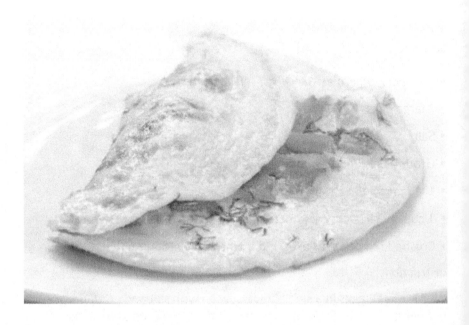

Egg Muffins

Ingredients - Allergies: SF, GF, DF, NF

Serving: 8 muffins

- 8 eggs
- 1 cup diced green bell pepper
- 1 cup diced onion
- 1 cup spinach
- 1/4 tsp. salt
- 1/8 tsp. ground black pepper
- 2 tbsp. water

Instructions

Heat the oven to 350 degrees F. Oil 8 muffin cups. Beat eggs together. Mix in bell pepper, spinach, onion, salt, black pepper, and water. Pour the mixture into muffin cups. Bake in the oven until muffins are done in the middle.

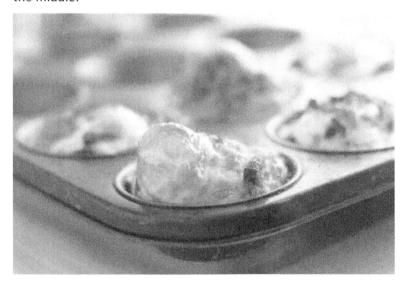

Smoked Salmon Scrambled Eggs

Ingredients, serves 2 - Allergies: SF, GF, DF, NF

- 1 tsp coconut oil
- 4 eggs
- 1 Tbs water
- 4 oz smoked salmon, sliced
- 1/2 avocado
- ground black pepper, to taste
- 4 chives, minced (or use 1 green onion, thinly sliced)

Instructions

Heat a skillet over medium heat. Add coconut oil to pan when hot. Meanwhile, scramble eggs. Add eggs to the hot skillet, along with smoked salmon. Stirring continuously, cook eggs until soft and fluffy. Remove from heat. Top with avocado, black pepper, and chives to serve.

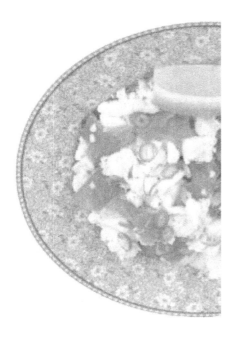

Steak and Eggs

Serves 2

Ingredients - Allergies: SF, GF, DF, NF

- 1/2 lb boneless beef steak or pork tenderloin
- 1/4 tsp ground black pepper
- 1/4 tsp sea salt (optional)
- 2 tsp coconut oil
- 1/4 onion, diced
- 1 red bell pepper, diced
- 1 handful spinach or arugula
- 2 eggs

Instructions

Season sliced steak or pork tenderloin with sea salt and black pepper. Heat a sauté pan over high heat. Add 1 tsp coconut oil, onions, and meat when pan is hot, and sauté until steak is slightly cooked. Add spinach and red bell pepper, and cook until steak is done to your liking. Meanwhile, heat a small fry pan over medium heat. Add remaining coconut oil, and fry two eggs. Top each steak with a fried egg to serve.

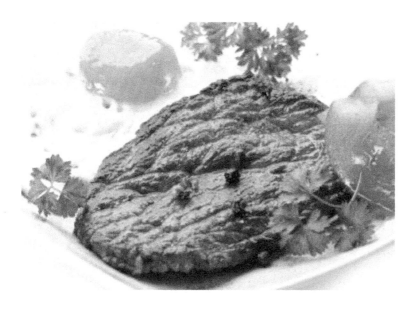

Broccoli Frittata

Serves 1

Ingredients - Allergies: SF, GF, DF, NF

- 2 large eggs
- Salt
- Ground black pepper
- 1 tsp. olive oil or avocado oil
- 1 cup Broccoli

Instructions

Whisk 2 large eggs in a small bowl. Season with salt and ground black pepper and set aside. Heat 1 tsp. olive oil in a medium skillet over medium heat. Add broccoli and cook, tossing, approx. 4-5 minutes. Add eggs; cook, stirring occasionally, until just set.

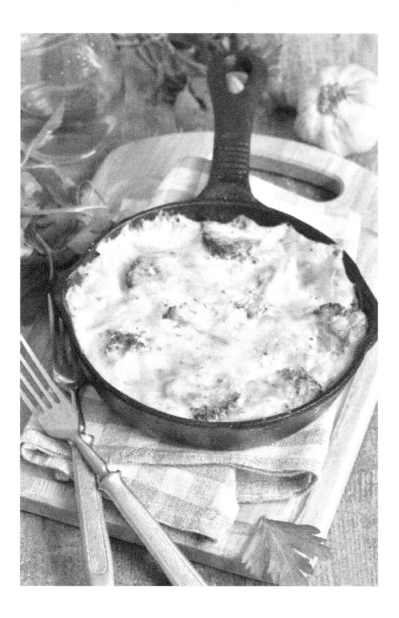

Mushrooms Omelet

Ingredients - Allergies: SF, GF, DF, NF

- 2 large eggs

- Salt

- Ground black pepper

- 1 tsp. <u>olive</u> oil or <u>avocado</u> oil

- 1 cup mushrooms

Instructions

Whisk 2 large eggs in a small bowl. Season with salt and ground black pepper and set aside. Heat 1 tsp. olive oil in a medium skillet over medium heat. Add mushrooms and cook, tossing, until slightly wilted (Approx. 3 minutes). Set aside. Add eggs and cook until set. Add mushrooms on top of the eggs. Flip eggs over mushrooms.

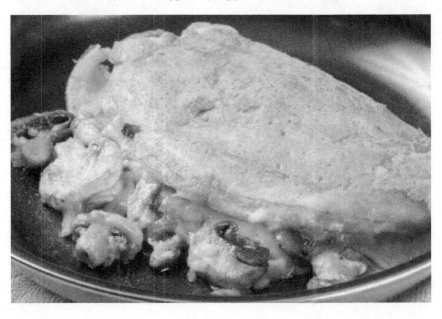

Broccoli, Red Peppers &Mushrooms Omelet

Ingredients - Allergies: SF, GF, DF, NF

- 2 large eggs

- Salt

- Ground black pepper

- 1 tsp. olive oil or avocado oil

- 1/2 cup broccoli

- 1/2 cup red peppers and mushrooms

Instructions

Whisk 2 large eggs in a small bowl. Season with salt and ground black pepper and set aside. Heat 1 tsp. olive oil in a medium skillet over medium heat. Add all veggies and cook, tossing, until slightly wilted (Approx. 3 minutes). Set aside. Add eggs and cook until set. Add veggies on top of the eggs. Flip eggs over veggies.

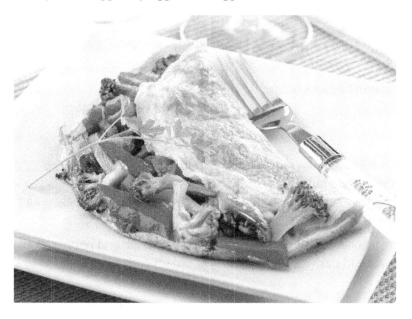

Spinach Egg Bake

Ingredients - Allergies: SF, GF, DF, NF

Serves 6

- 2 cups chopped red peppers or spinach
- 1 cup zucchini
- 2 tbsp. coconut oil
- 1 cup sliced mushrooms
- 1/2 cup sliced green onions
- 8 eggs
- 1 cup coconut milk
- 1/2 cup almond flour
- 2 tbsp. minced fresh parsley
- 1/2 tsp. dried basil
- 1/2 tsp. salt
- 1/4 tsp. ground black pepper

Instructions

Preheat oven to 350 degrees F. Put coconut oil in a skillet. Heat it to medium heat. Add mushrooms, onions, zucchini and red pepper (or spinach) until vegetables are tender, about 5 minutes. Drain veggies and spread them over the baking dish.

Beat eggs in a bowl with milk, flour, parsley, basil, salt, and pepper. Pour egg mixture into baking dish.

Bake in preheated oven until the center is set (approx. 35 to 40 minutes).

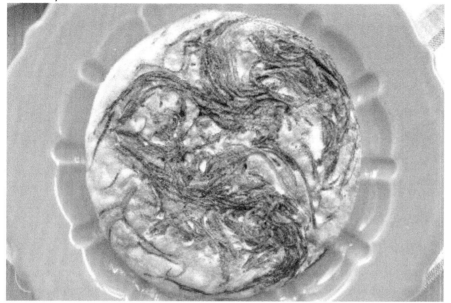

Spinach Frittata

6 servings

Ingredients - Allergies: SF, GF, DF, NF

- 2 tbsp. <u>olive</u> oil or <u>avocado</u> oil
- 1 Zucchini, sliced
- 1 cup torn fresh spinach
- 2 tbsp. sliced green onions
- 1 tsp. crushed garlic, salt and pepper to taste
- 1/3 cup coconut milk
- 6 eggs

Instructions

Heat olive oil in a skillet over medium heat. Add zucchini and cook until tender. Mix in spinach, green onions, and garlic. Season with salt and pepper. Continue cooking until spinach is wilted.

In a separate bowl, beat together eggs and coconut milk. Pour into the skillet over the vegetables. Reduce heat to low, cover, and cook until eggs are firm (5 to 7 minutes).

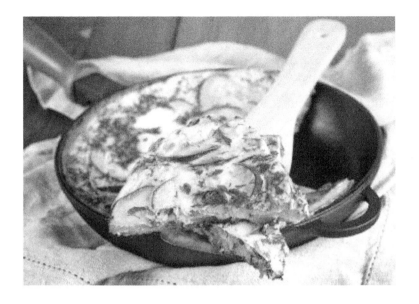

Superfoods Naan / Pancakes / Crepes

Ingredients - Allergies: SF, GF, DF, EF, V

- 1/2 cup <u>almond</u> flour

- 1/2 cup Tapioca Flour

- 1 cup Coconut Milk

- Salt

- <u>coconut</u> oil

Instructions

Mix all the ingredients together.

Heat a pan over medium heat and pour batter to desired thickness. Once the batter looks firm, flip it over to cook the other side.

If you want this to be a dessert crepe or pancake, then omit the salt. You can add minced garlic or ginger in the batter if you want, or some spices.

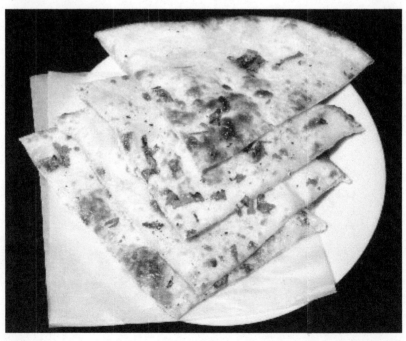

Frittata with Broccoli and Tomato

Serves 1

Ingredients - Allergies: SF, GF, DF, NF

- 2 large eggs
- Salt
- Ground black pepper
- 1 tsp. olive oil or cumin oil
- 1/2 cup broccoli & 1/2 cup sliced tomatoes
- Crushed red pepper flakes and a 1 Tbsp. chopped chives (optional)

Instructions

Whisk 2 large eggs in a small bowl. Season with salt and ground black pepper and set aside. Heat 1 tsp. oil in a medium skillet over medium heat. Add broccoli and tomatoes and cook, tossing, approx. 1 minute. Add eggs; cook, stirring occasionally, until just set, about 1 minute. Sprinkle with crushed red pepper flakes and chives.

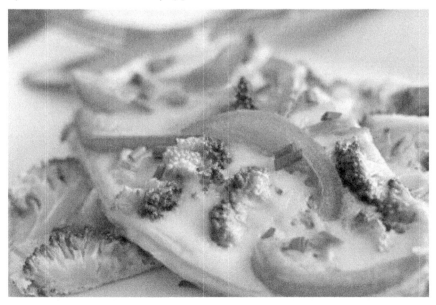

Frittata with Green and Red Peppers

Serves 1

Ingredients - Allergies: SF, GF, DF, NF

- 2 large eggs

- Salt

- Ground black pepper

- 1 tsp. olive oil or avocado oil

- 1/2 cup each chopped green and red peppers

Instructions

Whisk 2 large eggs in a small bowl. Season with salt and ground black pepper and set aside. Heat 1 tsp. olive oil in a medium skillet over medium heat. Add peppers and cook, tossing approx. 1 minute. Add eggs; cook, stirring occasionally, until just set, about 1 minute.

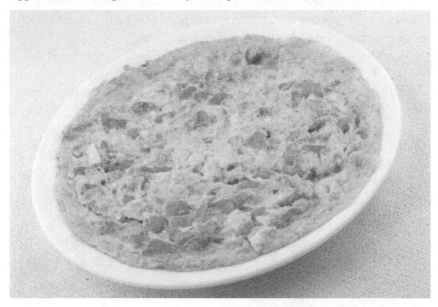

Eggs in Purgatory

Serves 1

Ingredients - Allergies: SF, GF, DF, NF

- 2 large eggs
- Salt
- 1 clove garlic, chopped.
- 1 tsp. olive oil or avocado oil
- 1 cup chopped tomatoes
- 1 Tbsp. hot red pepper flakes and 1 Tbsp. cilantro

Instructions

Heat 1 tsp. oil in a medium skillet over medium heat. Add garlic, chopped tomatoes and red pepper flakes and cook, tossing approx. 15 minutes. Add eggs and cook until eggs are done. Sprinkle with salt and cilantro.

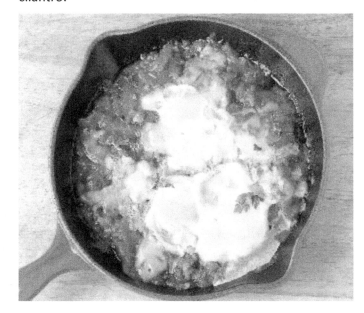

Frittata with Carrots, Green Peas and Asparagus
Serves 1

Ingredients - Allergies: SF, GF, DF, NF

- 2 large eggs
- Salt
- Ground black pepper
- 1 tsp. olive oil or avocado oil
- 1/2 cup cooked green peas
- 1/2 cup chopped carrot
- 1/2 cup asparagus
- 1 tbsp. fresh dill

Instructions

Whisk 2 large eggs in a small bowl. Season with salt and ground black pepper and set aside. Heat 1 tsp. oil in a medium skillet over medium heat. Add carrots and asparagus and cook, tossing, approx. 5 minutes. Add cooked and drained green peas. Add eggs; cook, stirring occasionally, until just set, about 1 minute. Sprinkle with dill.

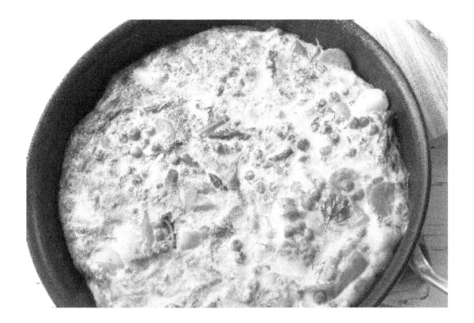

Zucchini Scrambled Eggs

Ingredients, serves 2 - Allergies: SF, GF, DF, NF

- 1 tsp coconut oil
- 4 eggs
- 1 Tbs water
- 1 zucchini, sliced
- ground black pepper, to taste

Instructions

Whisk 4 large eggs in a small bowl. Season with salt and ground black pepper and set aside. Heat 1 tsp. olive oil in a medium skillet over medium heat. Add sliced zucchini and cook, tossing, until wilted (Approx. 3 minutes). Set aside. Add eggs and cook until set, stirring occasionally. Serve with zucchini on a side.

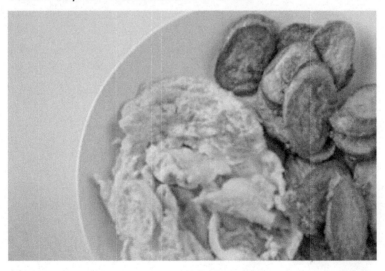

Frittata with Asparagus and Tomato

Serves 1

Ingredients - Allergies: SF, GF, DF, NF

- 2 large eggs
- Salt
- Ground black pepper
- 1 tsp. olive oil or avocado oil
- 1 cup asparagus
- 1/2 cup sliced tomatoes

Instructions

Whisk 2 large eggs in a small bowl. Season with salt and ground black pepper and set aside. Heat 1 tsp. oil in a medium skillet over medium heat. Add asparagus and cook, tossing approx. 4-5 minutes. Add tomatoes and eggs and cook, stirring occasionally, until just set, about 1 minute. Sprinkle with dill (optional).

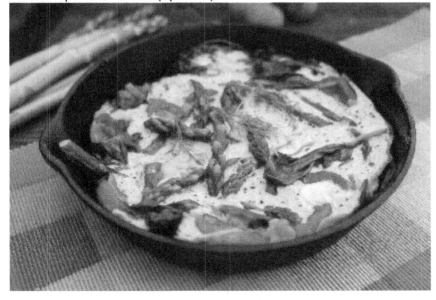

Eggs with Zucchini, Onions and Tomato
Serves 1

Ingredients - Allergies: SF, GF, DF, NF

- 2 large eggs
- Salt
- Ground black pepper
- 1 tsp. olive oil or avocado oil
- 1/3 cup sliced zucchini
- 1/3 cup chopped onions
- 1/3 cup sliced tomato
- Crushed red pepper flakes and a pinch of dill (optional)

Instructions

Whisk 2 large eggs in a small bowl. Season with salt and ground black pepper and set aside. Heat 1 tsp. olive oil in a medium skillet over medium heat. Add zucchini, onions and tomatoes and cook, tossing, until wilted (approx. 3-4 minutes). Add eggs and cook until just set.

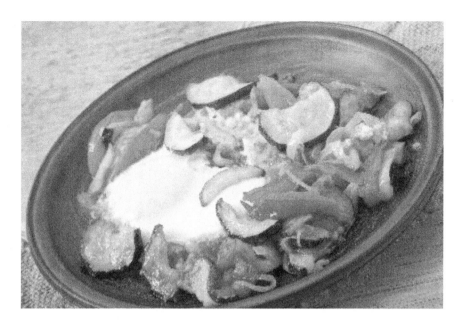

Frittata with Tomatoes and Spinach

Serves 1

Ingredients - Allergies: SF, GF, DF, NF

- 2 large eggs
- Salt
- Ground black pepper
- 1 tsp. olive oil or avocado oil
- 1/2 cup sliced tomatoes
- 1/3 cup spinach

Instructions

Whisk 2 large eggs in a small bowl. Season with salt and ground black pepper and set aside. Heat 1 tsp. olive oil in a medium skillet over medium heat. Add baby spinach and tomatoes and cook, tossing, until wilted (Approx. 1 minute). Add eggs; cook, stirring occasionally, until just set, about 1 minute.

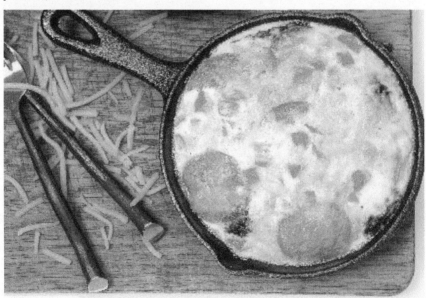

Zucchini Pancakes

Serves 3

Ingredients - Allergies: SF, GF, DF

- 2 medium zucchini
- 2 tbsp. chopped onion
- 3 beaten eggs
- 6 to 8 tbsp. almond flour
- 1 tsp. salt
- 1/2 tsp. ground black pepper
- coconut oil

Instructions

Heat the oven to 300 degrees F.

Grate the zucchini into a bowl and stir in the onion and eggs. Stir in 6 tbsp. of the flour, salt, and pepper.

Heat a large sauté pan over medium heat and add coconut oil in the pan. When the oil is hot, lower the heat to medium-low and add batter into the pan. Cook the pancakes about 2 minutes on each side, until browned. Place the pancakes in the oven.

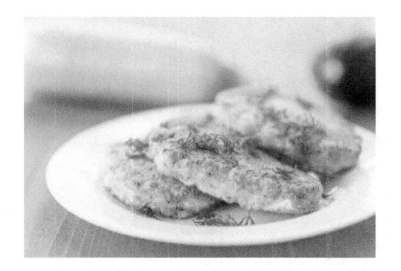

Eggs with Bok Choy

Serves 1

Ingredients - Allergies: SF, GF, DF, NF

- 2 large eggs
- Salt
- Ground black pepper
- 1 tsp. olive oil or avocado oil
- 1 cup bok choy

Instructions

Heat 1 tsp. olive oil in a medium skillet over medium heat. Add bok choy and cook, tossing, until wilted (Approx. 1 minute). Remove bok choy, add eggs and fry until done. Serve with bok choy.

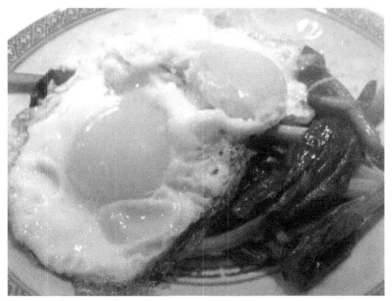

Chickpeas, Kale, Tomatoes Eggs

Serves 1

Ingredients - Allergies: SF, GF, DF, NF

- 2 large eggs
- Salt
- Ground black pepper
- 1 tsp. olive oil or avocado oil
- 1/3 cup sliced tomatoes
- 1/3 cup kale
- 1 cup cooked chickpeas

Instructions

Heat 1 tsp. olive oil in a medium skillet over medium heat. Add kale, tomatoes and chickpeas and cook, tossing, until kale wilts (Approx.3-4 minutes). Remove kale, chickpeas and tomatoes and season with sat and pepper. Fry eggs until done. Serve with kale, chickpeas and tomatoes.

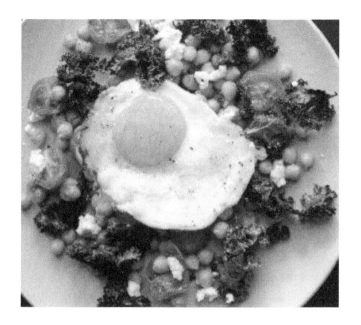

Leeks, Spinach, Eggs & Yogurt

Serves 1

Ingredients - Allergies: SF, GF, DF, NF

- 2 large eggs
- Salt
- Ground black pepper
- 1 tsp. olive oil or avocado oil
- 1/2 cup sliced leeks
- 1/3 cup spinach
- 1/3 cup thick Greek yogurt

Instructions

Heat 1 tsp. olive oil in a medium skillet over medium heat. Add leeks and coook for 5 minutes. Add spinach, salt and pepper and cook, tossing, until wilted (Approx. 1 minute). Break eggs on top and fry until done. Top with yogurt.

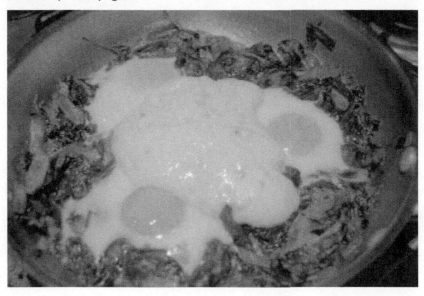

Chickpea Baked Eggs

Serves 2

Ingredients - Allergies: SF, GF, DF, NF

- 4 large eggs
- 1 cup cooked chickpeas
- Salt& Ground black pepper
- 1 tsp. olive oil
- 1/2 cup sliced onions & 1/2 cup sliced tomatoes
- 1 chopped garlic clove and 1/2cup. chopped spinach

Instructions

Saute onions, garlic and tomatoes for 5 minutes and then add chickpeas and spices. Saute for aminute longer, pour into small casserole dish, break eggs on top of it and cover with spinach. Baje in the oven until eggs are set.

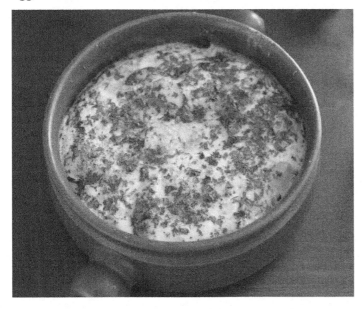

Asparagus Frittata

Serves 2

Ingredients - Allergies: SF, GF, DF, NF

- 2 large eggs
- Salt
- Ground black pepper
- 1 tsp. olive oil or cumin oil
- 1/2 cup broccoli & 1/2 cup sliced tomatoes

Instructions

Whisk 2 large eggs in a small bowl. Season with salt and ground black pepper and set aside. Heat 1 tsp. oil in a medium skillet over medium heat. Add asparagus and cook, tossing, approx. 3 minute. Add eggs; cook, stirring occasionally, until just set, about 1 minute.

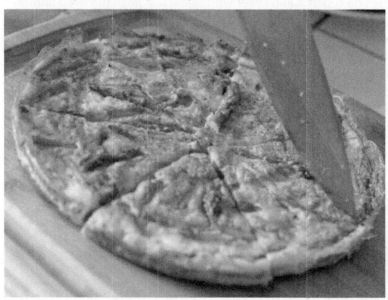

Brussels sprouts Frittata

Serves 2

Ingredients - Allergies: SF, GF, DF, NF

- 2 large eggs

- Salt

- Ground black pepper

- 1 tsp. olive oil or cumin oil

- 1 cup

Instructions

Whisk 2 large eggs in a small bowl. Season with salt and ground black pepper and set aside. Heat 1 tsp. oil in a medium skillet over medium heat. Add Brussels sprouts and cook, tossing, approx. 10 minute (until they get soft). Add eggs; cook, stirring occasionally, until just set, about 1 minute.

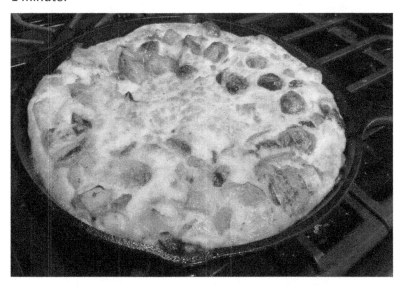

Zucchini Frittata

Serves 2

Ingredients - Allergies: SF, GF, DF, NF

- 2 large eggs
- Salt
- Ground black pepper
- 1 tsp. olive oil or cumin oil
- 1/2 cup sliced zucchinis

Instructions

Whisk 2 large eggs in a small bowl. Season with salt and ground black pepper and set aside. Heat 1 tsp. oil in a medium skillet over medium heat. Add zucchini and cook, tossing, approx. 3 minute. Add eggs; cook, stirring occasionally, until just set, about 1 minute.

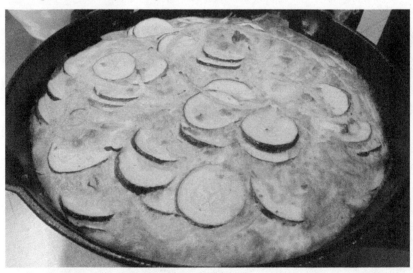

Tomato & Spring Onions Omelet

Serves 2

Ingredients - Allergies: SF, GF, DF, NF

- 2 large eggs
- Salt
- Ground black pepper
- 1 tsp. olive oil or cumin oil
- 1/2 cup quartered cherry tomatoes & 1/2 cup sliced mushrooms
- 1/2 cup sliced spring onions

Instructions

Whisk 2 large eggs in a small bowl. Season with salt and ground black pepper and set aside. Heat 1 tsp. oil in a medium skillet over medium heat. Add all veggies and cook, tossing, approx. 3 minute. Add eggs; cook, stirring occasionally, until just set, about 1 minute.

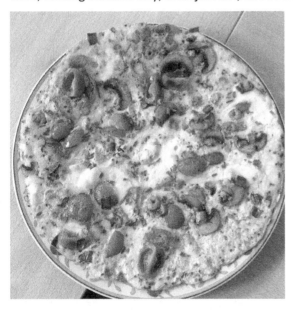

Kookoo Sabzi Herbs Frittata

Serves 2-3

Ingredients - Allergies: SF, GF, DF, NF

- 1/2 cup chopped parsley
- 1/4 cup chopped cilantro
- 1/4 cup chopped walnuts
- 4 large eggs
- 1/4 cup coconut milk
- 3/4 tsp. salt
- 1/2 cup chopped leeks
- 1/2 cup chopped spinach
- 1/4 cup chopped dill
- 1/4 tsp. freshly ground black pepper
- 1 tbsp. almond flour

Instructions

Whisk 4 large eggs in a bowl. Season with salt and ground black pepper, add coconut milk and almond flour, whisk a little bit more and set aside. Heat 1 tsp. oil in a medium skillet over medium heat. Add leeks and cook, tossing, approx. 3 minute. Add other veggies, walnuts and herbs to the eggs mixture, pour over leeks and cook, stirring occasionally, until just set, about 6-10 minutes.

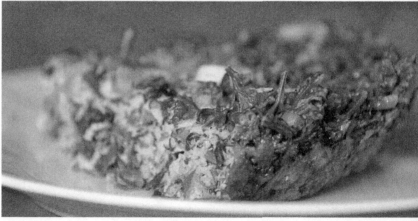

Cherry Tomato Frittata

Serves 2

Ingredients - Allergies: SF, GF, DF, NF

- 2 large eggs
- Salt
- Ground black pepper
- 1 tsp. olive oil or cumin oil
- 1/2 cup halved cherry tomatoes

Instructions

Whisk 2 large eggs in a small bowl. Season with salt and ground black pepper and set aside. Heat 1 tsp. oil in a medium skillet over medium heat. Add tomatoes and cook, tossing, approx. 2 minute. Add eggs; cook, stirring occasionally, until just set, about 1 minute.

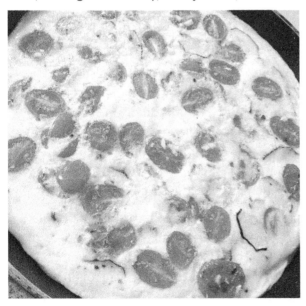

Savory Superfoods Pie Crust

Ingredients - Allergies: SF, GF, DF

- 11/4 cups blanched almond flour
- 1/3 cup tapioca flour
- 3/4 tsp. finely ground sea salt
- 3/4 tsp. paprika
- 1/2 tsp. ground cumin
- 1/8 tsp. ground white pepper
- 1/4 cup coconut oil
- 1 large egg

Instructions

Instructions

Place almond flour, tapioca flour, sea salt, vanilla, egg and coconut sugar (if you use coconut sugar) in the bowl of a food processor. Process 2-3 times to combine. Add oil and raw honey (if you use raw honey) and pulse with several one-second pulses and then let the food processor run until the mixture comes together. Move dough onto a plastic wrap sheet. Wrap and then press the dough into a 9-inch disk. Refrigerate for 30 minutes.

Remove plastic wrap. Press dough onto the bottom and up the sides of a 9-inch buttered pie dish. Crimp a little bit the edges of crust. Cool in the refrigerator for 20 minutes. Put the oven rack to middle position and preheat oven to 375F. Put in the oven and bake until golden brown.

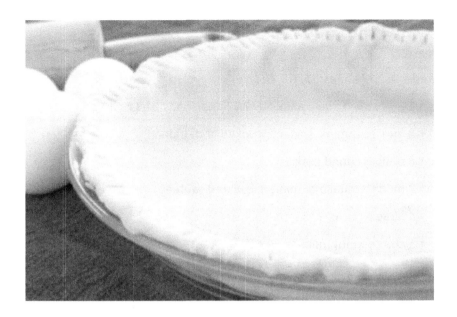

Spinach Quiche

Serves 2-3

Ingredients - Allergies: SF, GF, DF, NF

- 1 Precooked and cooled Savory Superfoods Pie Crust

- 8 ounces organic spinach, cooked and drained

- 6 ounces cubed pork

- 2 medium shallots, thinly sliced and sautéed

- 4 large eggs

- 1 cup coconut milk

- 3/4 tsp. salt

- 1/4 tsp. freshly ground black pepper

Instructions

Brown the pork in coconut oil and then add the spinach and shallots. Set aside once done.

Preheat oven to 350F. In a large bowl, combine eggs, milk, salt and pepper. Whisk until foamy. Add in about 3/4 of the drained filling mixture, reserving the other 1/4 to "top" the quiche. Pour egg mixture into crust and place remaining filling on top of the quiche.

Place quiche in oven in the center of the middle rack and bake undisturbed for 45 to 50 minutes.

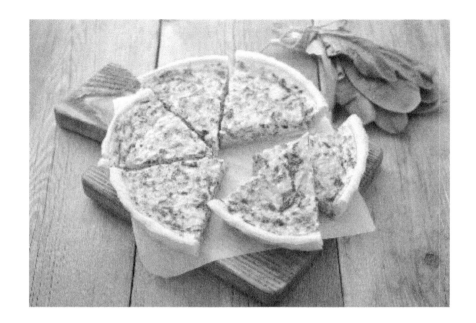

Mushroom Quiche

Serves 2-3

Ingredients - Allergies: SF, GF, DF, NF

- 1 Precooked and cooled Savory Superfoods Pie Crust
- 1 cup sliced mushrooms
- 6 ounces cubed pork
- 2 medium shallots, thinly sliced and sautéed
- 4 large eggs
- 1 cup coconut milk
- 3/4 tsp. salt
- 1/4 tsp. freshly ground black pepper

Instructions

Brown the pork in coconut oil and then add the mushrooms and shallots. Set aside once done.

Preheat oven to 350F. In a large bowl, combine eggs, milk, salt and pepper. Whisk until foamy. Add in about 3/4 of the drained filling mixture, reserving the other 1/4 to "top" the quiche. Pour egg mixture into crust and place remaining filling on top of the quiche.

Place quiche in oven in the center of the middle rack and bake undisturbed for 45 to 50 minutes.

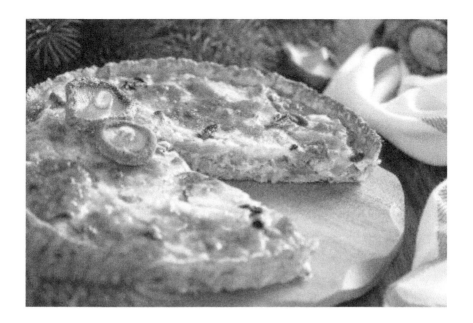

Tomato Quiche

Serves 2-3

Ingredients - Allergies: SF, GF, DF, NF

- 1 Precooked and cooled Savory Superfoods Pie Crust
- 1 cup sliced tomatoes
- 6 ounces cubed pork
- 2 medium shallots, thinly sliced and sautéed
- 4 large eggs
- 1 cup coconut milk
- 3/4 tsp. salt
- 1/4 cup. arugula
- 1/4 tsp. freshly ground black pepper

Instructions

Brown the pork and shallots in the coconut oil. Set aside once done.

Preheat oven to 350F. In a large bowl, combine eggs, milk, salt and pepper. Whisk until foamy. Add in about 3/4 of the drained filling mixture and tomatoes, reserving the other 1/4 to "top" the quiche. Pour egg mixture into crust and place remaining filling on top of the quiche.

Place quiche in oven in the center of the middle rack and bake undisturbed for 45 to 50 minutes. Sprinkle with arugula.

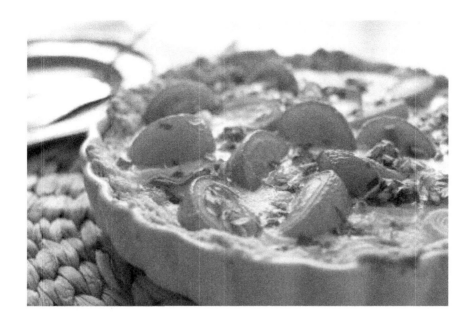

Vegetarian Tomato Quiche

Serves 2-3

Ingredients - Allergies: SF, GF, DF, NF

- 1 Precooked and cooled Savory Superfoods Pie Crust
- 2 cups sliced tomatoes
- 4 large eggs
- 1 cup coconut milk
- 3/4 tsp. salt
- 1/4 cup. Fresh basil
- 1/4 tsp. freshly ground black pepper

Instructions

Preheat oven to 350F. In a large bowl, combine eggs, milk, salt and pepper. Whisk until foamy. Pour egg mixture into crust and place sliced tomatoes on top of the quiche.

Place quiche in oven in the center of the middle rack and bake undisturbed for 45 to 50 minutes. Sprinkle with basil.

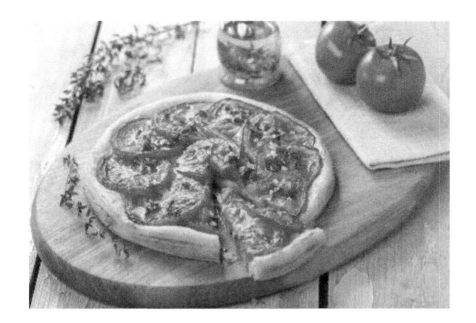

Onions & Swiss Chard Quiche

Serves 2-3

Ingredients - Allergies: SF, GF, DF, NF

- 1 Precooked and cooled Savory Superfoods Pie Crust
- 2 cups chopped Swiss Chard
- 4 large eggs
- 1 cup coconut milk
- 3/4 tsp. salt
- 1 cup chopped onions
- 1/4 tsp. freshly ground black pepper

Instructions

Preheat oven to 350F. In a large bowl, combine eggs, milk, salt and pepper. Whisk until foamy. Put Swiss chard and onions in the crust. Pour egg mixture over veggies in the crust.

Place quiche in oven in the center of the middle rack and bake undisturbed for 45 to 50 minutes.

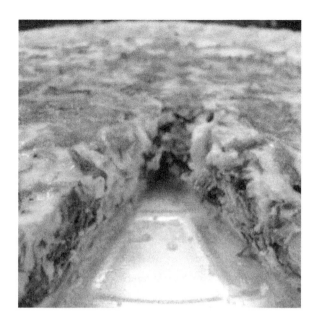

Eggplant Quiche

Serves 2-3

Ingredients - Allergies: SF, GF, DF, NF

- 1 Precooked and cooled Savory Superfoods Pie Crust
- 2 cups cubed eggplant
- 4 large eggs
- 1 cup coconut milk
- 3/4 tsp. salt
- 1/4 tsp. freshly ground black pepper

Instructions

Preheat oven to 350F. In a large bowl, combine eggs, milk, salt and pepper. Whisk until foamy. Put eggplant in the crust. Pour egg mixture over eggplant in the crust.

Place quiche in oven in the center of the middle rack and bake undisturbed for 45 to 50 minutes.

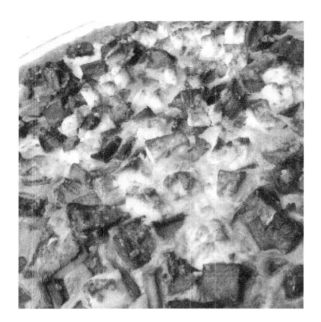

Dandelion Olives Quiche

Serves 2-3

Ingredients - Allergies: SF, GF, DF, NF

- 1 Precooked and cooled Savory Superfoods Pie Crust
- 2 cups chopped dandelion leaves
- 4 large eggs
- 1 cup coconut milk
- 3/4 tsp. salt
- 3/4 cup sliced pitted olives
- 1/4 tsp. freshly ground black pepper

Instructions

Preheat oven to 350F. In a large bowl, combine eggs, milk, salt and pepper. Whisk until foamy. Put dandelion and olives in the crust. Pour egg mixture over veggies in the crust.

Place quiche in oven in the center of the middle rack and bake undisturbed for 45 to 50 minutes.

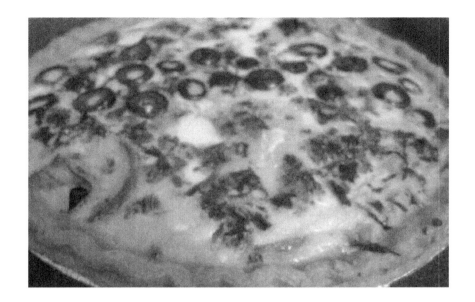

Carrot Quiche

Serves 2-3

Ingredients - Allergies: SF, GF, DF, NF

- 1 Precooked and cooled Savory Superfoods Pie Crust
- 1 cup shredded carrot & 1 cup sliced leeks
- 2 carrots thinly sliced lengthwise for decoration
- 4 large eggs
- 1 cup coconut milk
- 3/4 tsp. salt & 1 tsp. dried rosemary
- 1/4 tsp. freshly ground black pepper

Instructions

Preheat oven to 350F. In a large bowl, combine eggs, milk, salt and pepper. Whisk until foamy. Put shredded carrots and leeks in the crust. Pour egg mixture over veggies in the crust and decorate with sliced carrots.

Place quiche in oven in the center of the middle rack and bake undisturbed for 45 to 50 minutes.

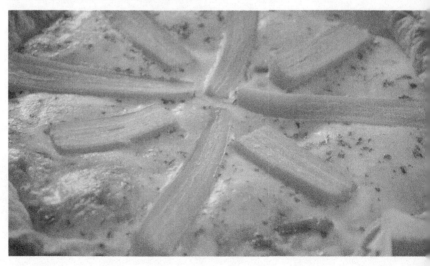

Swiss Chard & Leeks Quiche

Serves 2-3

Ingredients - Allergies: SF, GF, DF, NF

- 1 Precooked and cooled Savory Superfoods Pie Crust
- 2 cups chopped Swiss chard leaves
- 4 large eggs
- 1 cup coconut milk
- 3/4 tsp. salt
- 1 cup sliced leeks
- 1/4 tsp. freshly ground black pepper

Instructions

Preheat oven to 350F. In a large bowl, combine eggs, milk, salt and pepper. Whisk until foamy. Put Swiss chard and leeks in the crust. Pour egg mixture over veggies in the crust.

Place quiche in oven in the center of the middle rack and bake undisturbed for 45 to 50 minutes.

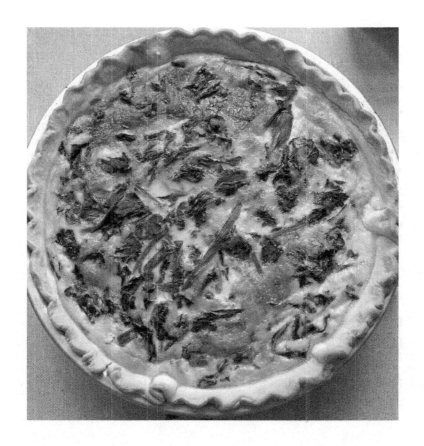

Cottage Cheese Sesame Balls

Ingredients - Allergies: SF, GF, EF

- 16 ounce farmers cheese or cottage cheese
- 1 cup finely chopped almonds
- 1and 1/2 cups oatmeal

In a large bowl, combine blended cottage cheese, almonds and oatmeal. Make balls and roll in sesame seeds mix.

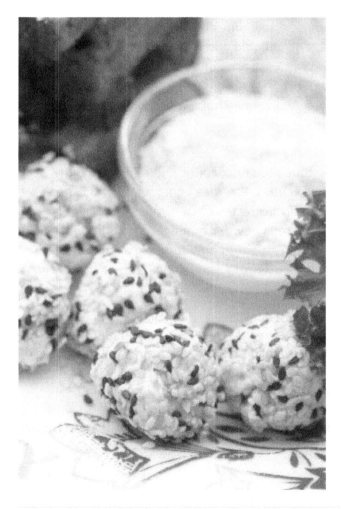

Superfoods Smoothies

Put the liquid in first. Surrounded by tea or yogurt, the blender blades can move freely. Next, add chunks of fruits or vegetables. Leafy greens are going into the pitcher last. Preferred liquid is green tea, but you can use almond or coconut milk or herbal tea.

Start slow. If your blender has speeds, start it on low to break up big pieces of fruit. Continue blending until you get a puree. If your blender can pulse, pulse a few times before switching to a puree mode. Once you have your liquid and fruit pureed, start adding greens, very slowly. Wait until previous batch of greens has been completely blended. I use Vitamix blenders because they're sturdy and offer 7 year warranty. That was definitely the best investment in my health.

Thicken? Added too much tea or coconut milk? Thicken your smoothie by adding ice cubes, flax meal, chia seeds or oatmeal. Once you get used to various tastes of smoothies, add any seaweed, spirulina, chlorella powder or ginger for additional kick. Experiment with any Superfoods in powder form at this point. Think of adding any nut butter or sesame paste too or some Superfoods oils.

Rotate! Rotate your greens; don't always drink the same smoothie! At the beginning try 2 different greens every week and later introduce third and fourth one weekly. And keep rotating them. Don't use spinach and kale all the time. Try beets greens, they have a pinch of pink in them and that add great color to your smoothie. Here is the list of leafy green for you to try: spinach, kale, dandelion, chards, beet leaves, arugula, lettuce, collard greens, bok choy, cabbage, cilantro, parsley.

Flavor! Flavor smoothies with ground vanilla bean, cinnamon, raw honey, nutmeg, cloves, almond butter, cayenne pepper, ginger or just about any seeds or chopped nuts combination.

Not only are green smoothies high in nutrients, vitamins and fiber, they can also make any vegetable you probably don't like (be it kale, spinach or broccoli) taste great. The secret behind blending the perfect smoothie is using sweet fruits or nuts or seeds to give your drink a unique taste.

There's a reason kale and spinach seem to be the main ingredients in almost every green smoothie. Not only do they give smoothies their verdant color, they are also packed with calcium, protein and iron.

Although blending alone increases the accessibility of carotenoids, since the presence of fats is known to increase carotenoid absorption from leafy greens, it is possible that coconut oil, nuts and seeds in a smoothie could increase absorption further.

Fruits and Veggies preparation

• Wash fruits and veggies

• Pluck leaves and stems from berries

• Core apples (optional)

• Peel orange, lemon, lime, grapefruit, kiwi, beet, pomegranate, ginger, dragon fruit and banana

• Peel and take the seeds out of papaya

• Remove seeds from peppers, apricots, peaches, cherries, plums and prunes

• Mangos, melons and avocados should be peeled, and inner seed taken out

• Watermelons should have their outer rind removed.

• Scoop out the flesh from passion fruit

• Cut fruits and veggies in 2-inch slices

If you can't find some ingredient, replace it with the closest one.

All details about each ingredient (vitamins, minerals, antioxidants etc.) can be found in my free Superfoods Reference book: http://www.SuperfoodsToday.com/FREE

Smoothies

Carrot Date Smoothie

2 Carrots

2 Apples

1 cup of crushed ice

Pinch of nutmeg

½ tsp. Cinnamon

2 dates

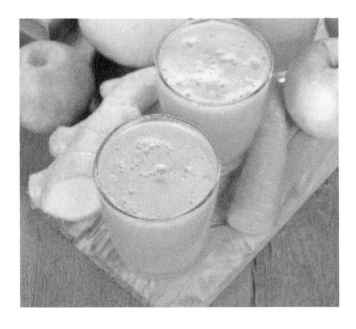

Watermelon Apple smoothie

- 1 cup Seedless Watermelon

- ½ cup Pomegranate

- 2 apples

- 1/2 cup Raspberries

- 1 tbsp. Maqui

- 1 cup Yerba Mate tea

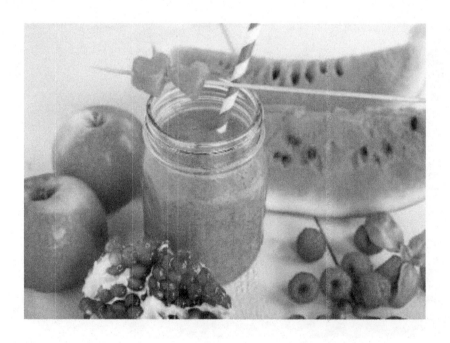

Watermelon Red Grapefruit Smoothie

- 1 cup seedless Watermelon

- 1 Red Grapefruit

- 1 cup red spinach

- 1 cup crushed ice

- 2 tablespoons ground flax seeds

- 1 tbsp. Bee Pollen

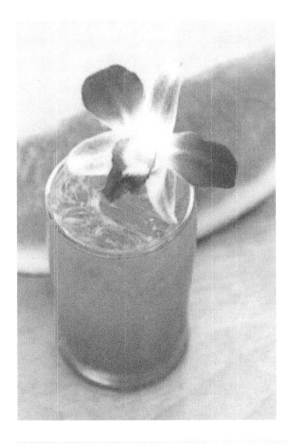

Strawberry Carrot Smoothie

- 1 cup frozen strawberries

- 1 banana

- 1 carrot

- 1 cup crushed ice

- 2 tablespoons Hemp seeds

- 1 tsp. Fresh Mint

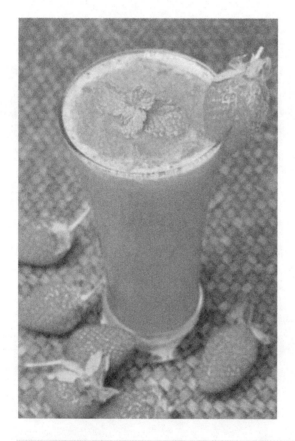

Strawberries Yogurt Smoothie

- 1 cup strawberries

- 1 cup low-fat plain yogurt

- 3 ice cubes

- 1 tbsp. Acai

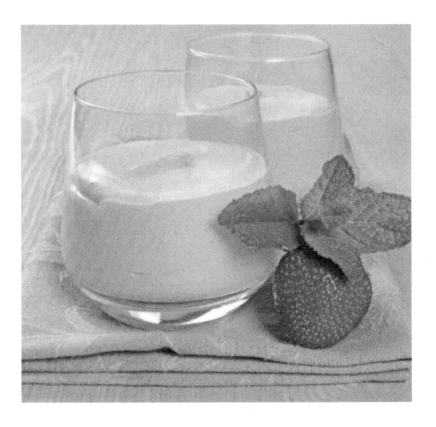

Frozen Berries Smoothie

1 cup frozen raspberries

1 cup frozen blueberries

1 cup of kefir

Pinch of nutmeg

1 tbsp. Minced ginger

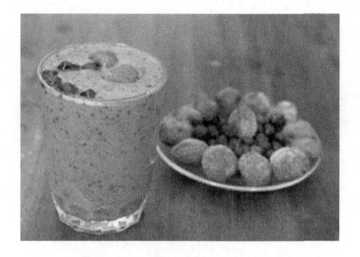

Superfoods Smoothie Popsicles

Green Layer: 2 Kiwis + 1 Granny Smith apple + 1 ice cube

Yellow Layer: 1 Mango + 1 Orange + 1 ice cube

Red Layer: 1 cup of seedless watermelon + 1/2 cup of Raspberries

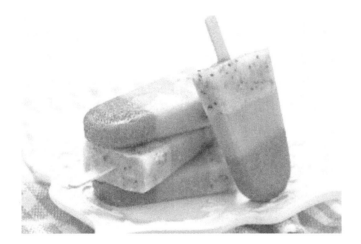

Pomegranate Watermelon Smoothie

1 cup seedless watermelon

1 cup Pomegranate seeds

1 cup of crushed ice

2 carrots

½ tsp. Mint

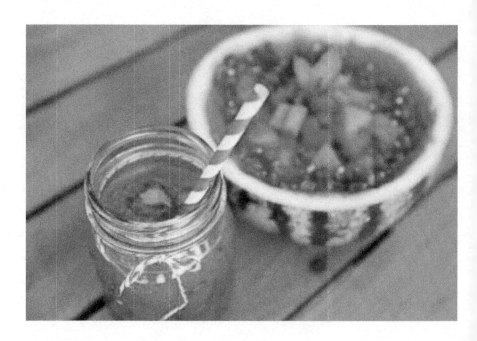

Orange Carrot Smoothie

2 Carrots

2 Oranges

1 cup of crushed ice

Pinch of cinnamon

1 tbsp. Minced ginger

1 tbsp. Chia seeds

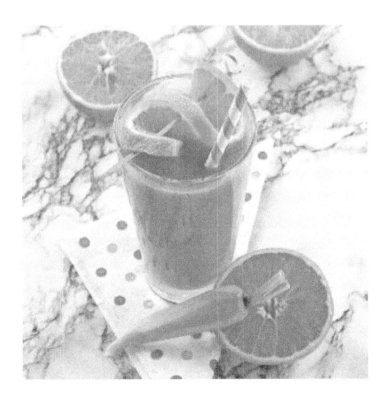

Carrot Orange Papaya Smoothie

2 Carrots

1 Papaya

1 Orange

1 cup of crushed ice

Pinch of nutmeg

½ tsp. Cinnamon

1 tsp. Bee Pollen

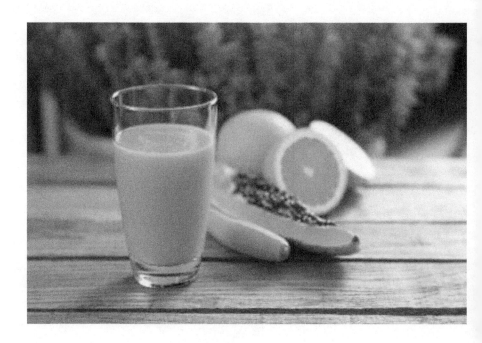

Berries Kefir Smoothie

1/2 cup blackberries

½ cup raspberries

1/2 cup of crushed ice

1 cup Kefir

1 tbsp. Chia seeds

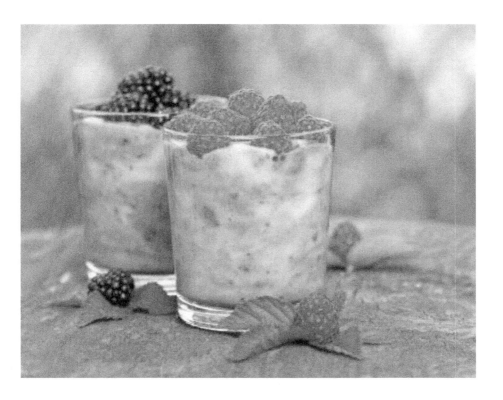

Red Currants Blueberry Smoothie

1 cup Spinach

1/2 cup blueberries

1/2 cup red currants

1 cup of crushed ice

Pinch of nutmeg

½ tsp. sesame seeds

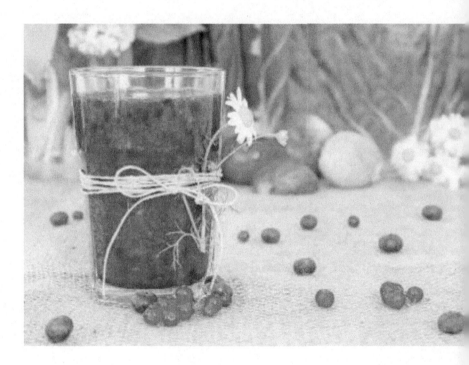

Blueberry Avocado Smoothie

- 1/2 avocado

- 1 cup spinach

- 1 cup blueberries, frozen

- 1 tsp. coconut oil

- 3/4 cup water

- 1 cup crushed ice

- Top with Cranberries

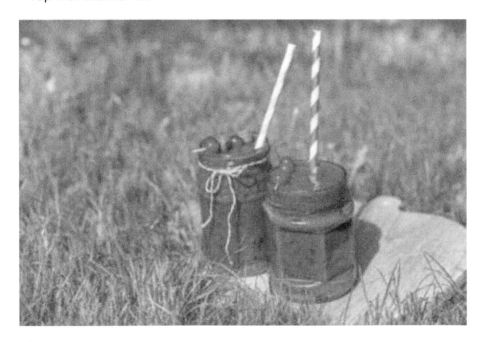

Blueberry Kefir & Spinach Smoothie

- 1 cup blueberries

- 1 cup chopped Cantaloupe

- 1 cup Red Spinach

- 1 cup Green tea

- 1 tbsp. Hemp seeds

- ½ tsp. Cinnamon

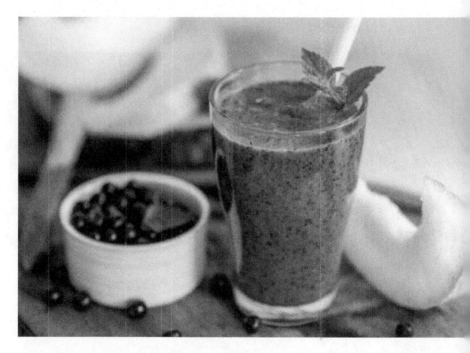

Blackberry Yogurt & Purple Carrots Smoothie

- 1 cup blueberries

- 2 purple carrots

- 1 cup Yogurt

- 1 tbsp. ground flax seeds

- Top with Blackberries

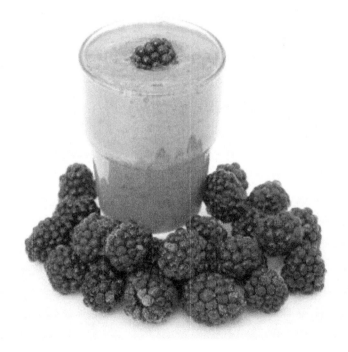

Blackberry Banana Smoothie

- 1 cup blueberries

- 1 banana

- 1 cup of crushed ice

- ½ tsp. Cinnamon

- Top with Blackberries and Banana

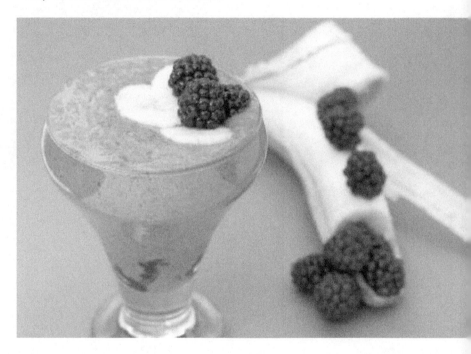

Coconut Chia Pudding

- 1/4 cup Chia seeds

- 1 cup coconut milk

- 1/2 tablespoon Royall jelly

- 1 tsp. Ground Vanilla Bean

- a pinch of Nutmeg

- Top with Blueberries

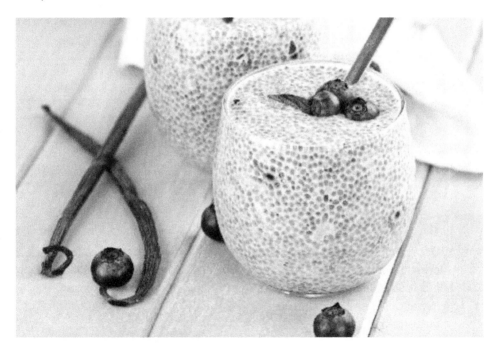

Salad Dressings

Italian Dressing

Serves 1 - Allergies: SF, GF, DF, EF, V, NF

- 1 tsp. olive oil or cumin oil
- lemon
- minced garlic
- salt
- 1 Tbsp. of Spirulina, Chlorella, Maca or Matcha (optional)

Yogurt Dressing

Serves 1 - Allergies: SF, GF, DF, EF, V, NF

- half a cup of plain low-fat Greek yogurt or low-fat buttermilk
- olive oil or avocado oil
- minced garlic
- salt
- lemon

Occasionally I would add a tsp. of mustard or some herbs like basil, oregano, marjoram, chives, thyme, parsley, dill or mint. If you like spicy hot food, add some cayenne in the dressing. It will speed up your metabolism and have interesting hot spicy effect in cold yogurt or buttermilk.

Salads

Large Fiber Loaded Salad with Italian Dressing

Serves 1 - Allergies: SF, GF, EF, NF

- 1 cup of spinach

- 1 cup of shredded cabbage, sauerkraut or lettuce. Cabbage has more substance.

- Italian or Yogurt dressing

- Cayenne pepper (optional)

- Few sprigs of cilantro (optional)

- 2 spring (green) onions (optional)

Nutrition Facts

Serving Size 105 g

Amount Per Serving

Calories 64	Calories from Fat 44

	% Daily Value*
Total Fat 4.9g	**7%**
Saturated Fat 0.7g	**4%**
Cholesterol 0mg	**0%**
Sodium 36mg	**2%**
Potassium 286mg	**8%**
Total Carbohydrates 5.1g	**2%**
Dietary Fiber 2.4g	**10%**
Sugars 2.4g	
Protein 1.8g	

Vitamin A 58%	•	Vitamin C 57%
Calcium 6%	•	Iron 6%

Nutrition Grade A

* Based on a 2000 calorie diet

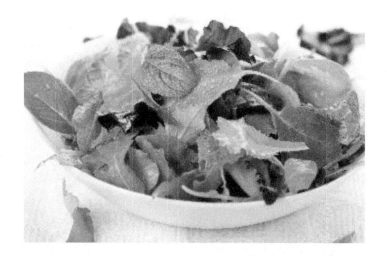

Large Fiber Loaded Salad with Yogurt Dressing

Serves 1 - Allergies: SF, GF, EF, NF

- 1 cup of spinach

- 1 cup of shredded cabbage or lettuce. Cabbage has more substance.

- Italian or Yogurt dressing

- Cayenne pepper (optional)

- Few sprigs of cilantro (optional)

- 2 spring (green) onions (optional)

Nutrition Facts

Serving Size 226 g

Amount Per Serving

Calories 136	Calories from Fat 40

	% Daily Value*
Total Fat 4.5g	**7%**
Saturated Fat 1.7g	**8%**
Cholesterol 7mg	**2%**
Sodium 122mg	**5%**
Potassium 573mg	**16%**
Total Carbohydrates 13.8g	**5%**
Dietary Fiber 2.4g	**10%**
Sugars 11.0g	
Protein 8.7g	

Vitamin A 59%	•	Vitamin C 58%
Calcium 28%	•	Iron 7%

Nutrition Grade A

* Based on a 2000 calorie diet

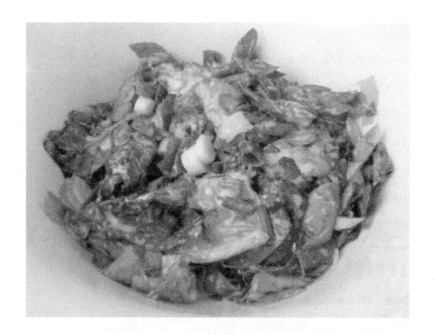

Large Fiber Loaded Salad as a meal on its own – only 258 calories per serving

Serves 1 - Allergies: SF, GF, EF, NF

This is what I eat every second evening and I can't get enough of it!!! This is the real secret to lose weight while having full stomach with grade A ingredients!!

- 1 cup of spinach

- 1 cup of shredded cabbage

- Yogurt dressing

- Cayenne pepper (optional)

- Few sprigs of cilantro (optional)

- 2 spring (green) onions

- 5 oz. low-fat farmers cheese

Pour yogurt dressing into the salad bowl. Add farmers' cheese and mix thoroughly. Cut spring onions in small pieces and add to the cheese mixture and mix. Add spinach and cabbage and mix thoroughly. Add spices (optional).

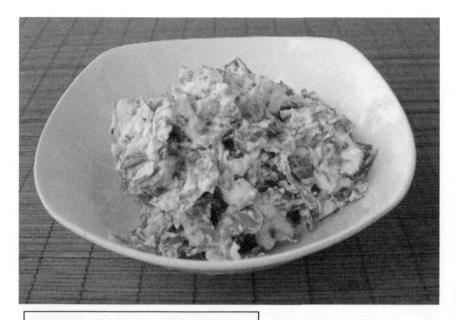

Nutrition Facts

Serving Size 401 g

Amount Per Serving

Calories 258   Calories from Fat 62

	% Daily Value*
Total Fat 6.8g	**11%**
Saturated Fat 2.0g	**10%**
Cholesterol 7mg	**2%**
Sodium 708mg	**30%**
Potassium 656mg	**19%**
Total Carbohydrates 21.5g	**7%**
Dietary Fiber 3.2g	**13%**
Sugars 15.9g	
Protein 26.6g	

Vitamin A 65%	•	Vitamin C 68%
Calcium 30%	•	Iron 9%

Nutrition Grade A-

* Based on a 2000 calorie diet

Greek Salad

Serves 4 - Allergies: SF, GF, EF, NF

- 1 head iceberg lettuce
- 1 head romaine lettuce
- 1 lb. plump tomatoes
- 6 oz. Greek or black olives, sliced
- 4 oz. sliced radishes
- 4 oz. low-fat feta or goat cheese
- 2 oz. anchovies (optional)

Dressing:
- 3 oz. olive oil or avocado oil
- 3 oz. fresh lemon juice
- 1 tsp. dried oregano
- 1 tsp. salt
- 4 cloves garlic, minced

Wash and cut lettuce into pieces. Slice tomatoes in quarters. Combine olives, lettuce, tomatoes, and radishes in large bowl. Mix dressing ingredients together and toss with vegetables. Pour out into a serving bowl. Crumble feta/goat cheese over all, and arrange anchovy fillets on top (if desired).

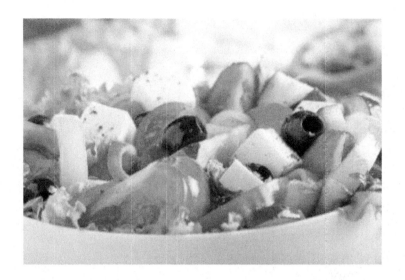

Almond, Quinoa, Red Peppers & Arugula Salad

Serves 2

Ingredients - Allergies: SF, GF, DF, EF, NF, V

- 1 cup cooked quinoa mixed with 1 tbsp. pumpkin seeds
- 1/2 cup chopped almonds
- 1 cup chopped arugula
- 1/2 cup sliced red peppers

Dressing:
- 1 tbsp. olive oil or cumin oil
- 1 tbsp. fresh lemon juice
- pinch of sea salt

Instructions: Mix all ingredients.

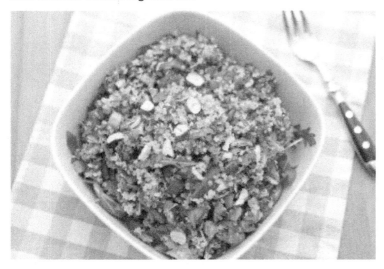

Asparagus, Quinoa & Red Peppers Salad

Serves 2

Ingredients - Allergies: SF, GF, DF, EF, NF, V

- 1 cup cooked quinoa mixed with 1 tbsp. sunflower seeds
- 1 cup sliced red peppers
- 1 cup grilled asparagus
- Garnish with lime and parsley

Dressing:
- 1 tbsp. olive oil or avocado oil
- 1 tbsp. fresh lemon juice
- pinch of sea salt

Instructions: Mix all ingredients.

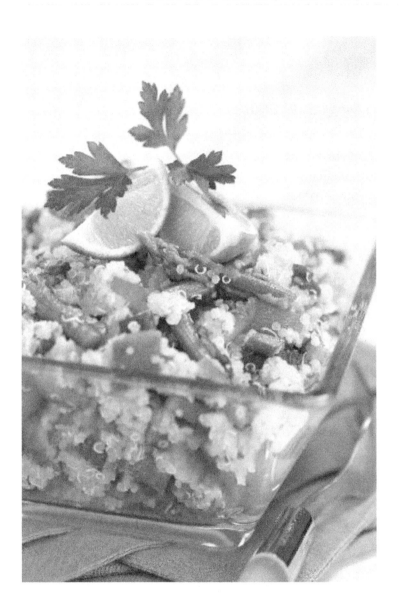

Chickpeas, Quinoa, Cucumber & Tomato Salad

Serves 2

Ingredients - Allergies: SF, GF, DF, EF, NF, V

- 1 cup cooked quinoa mixed with 1 tbsp. sesame seeds
- 1 cup cooked chickpeas
- 1 cup chopped cucumber and green onions
- 1/2 cup chopped tomato

Dressing:
- 1 tbsp. olive oil or avocado oil
- 1 tbsp. fresh lemon juice
- pinch of sea salt

Instructions: Mix all ingredients.

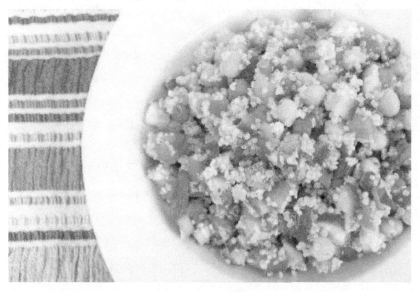

Strawberry Spinach Salad

Serves 4-6

Ingredients - Allergies: SF, GF, DF, EF, V

- 2 tbsp. black sesame seeds
- 1 tbsp. poppy seeds
- 1/2 cup olive oil or avocado oil
- 1/4 cup lemon juice
- 1/4 tsp. paprika
- 1 bag fresh spinach - chopped, washed and dried
- 1 quart strawberries, sliced
- 1/4 cup toasted slivered almonds

Instructions

Whisk together the sesame seeds, olive oil, poppy seeds, paprika, lemon juice and onion. Refrigerate.
In a large bowl, combine the spinach, strawberries and almonds. Pour dressing over salad. Toss and refrigerate 15 minutes before serving.

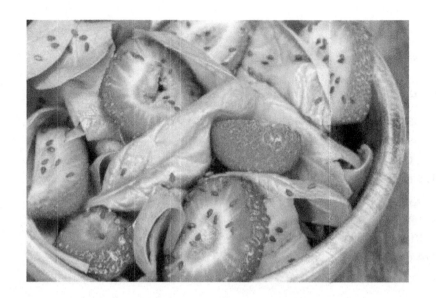

Tuna Bean Salad

Serves 1 - Allergies: SF, GF, DF, EF, NF

Ingredients

- 1 can tuna in water, drained
- 1/3 cup four bean mix (or just white or red beans), drained, rinsed
- 1 tomato, deseeded, chopped
- 1 large celery stick, trimmed, finely chopped
- 1/2 small onion, halved, thinly sliced
- 1/2 cup flat-leaf parsley leaves, chopped
- 1/2 lemon, rind finely grated, juiced
- 1 garlic clove, crushed & 1 tbsp. extra-virgin olive oil

Mix all ingredients and serve.

Nutrition Facts

Serving Size 335 g

Amount Per Serving

Calories 345   Calories from Fat 114

	% Daily Value*
Total Fat 12.6g	**19%**
Saturated Fat 2.3g	**11%**
Trans Fat 0.0g	
Cholesterol 28mg	**9%**
Sodium 115mg	**5%**
Potassium 1191mg	**34%**
Total Carbohydrates 27.1g	**9%**
Dietary Fiber 7.8g	**31%**
Sugars 6.1g	
Protein 31.5g	

Vitamin A 68%	•	Vitamin C 107%
Calcium 9%	•	Iron 29%

Nutrition Grade A

* Based on a 2000 calorie diet

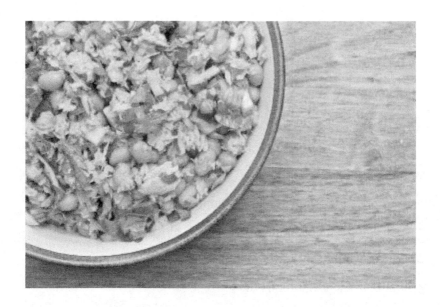

Greek Cucumber Salad
Serves 2-3

Ingredients - Allergies: SF, GF, EF, NF

- 2-3 cucumbers, sliced
- 2 teaspoons salt
- 3 tbsp. lemon juice
- 1/4 tsp. paprika
- 1/4 tsp. white pepper
- 1/2 clove garlic, minced
- 4 fresh green onions, diced
- 1 cup thick Greek Yogurt

- 1/4 tsp. paprika

Instructions

Slice cucumbers thinly, sprinkle with salt and mix. Set aside for one hour. Mix lemon juice, water, garlic, paprika and white pepper, and set aside. Squeeze liquid from cucumber slices a few at a time, and place slices in the bowl. Discard liquid. Add lemon juice mixture, green onions, and yogurt. Mix and sprinkle additional paprika or dill over top. Chill for 1-2 hours.

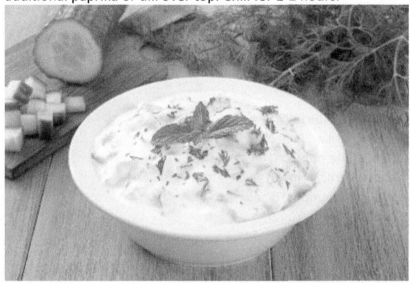

Mediterranean Salad

Serves 3-4

Ingredients - Allergies: SF, GF, DF, EF, V, NF

- 1 medium head romaine lettuce, torn
- 3 small tomatoes, diced
- 1 medium cucumber, sliced
- 1 small green bell pepper, sliced
- 1 small onion, cut into rings
- 6 radishes, thinly sliced
- 1/2 cup flat leaf parsley, chopped
- 1/3 cup olive oil or avocado oil
- 3 tbsp. lemon juice
- 1 garlic clove, minced
- Salt & pepper
- 1 tsp. fresh mint, minced

Instructions

Combine lettuce, tomatoes, cucumber, pepper, onion, radishes & parsley in a salad bowl. Whisk together olive oil, lemon juice, garlic, salt, pepper & mint. Pour over salad & toss to coat.

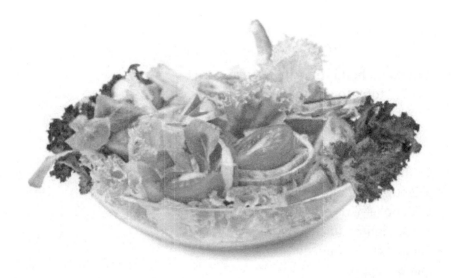

Pomegranate Avocado salad

Serves 1

Ingredients - Allergies: SF, GF, DF, EF, V

- 1 cup mixed greens, spinach, arugula, red leaf lettuce
- 1 ripe avocado, cut into 1/2-inch pieces
- 1/2 cup pomegranate seeds
- 1/4 cup pecan
- 1/4 cup blackberries
- 1/4 cup cherry tomatoes
- olive oil or avocado oil, salt, lemon juice

Instructions

Combine greens, pecan, cut avocado, tomatoes, pomegranates and blackberries in a salad bowl. Whisk together salt, olive oil and lemon juice and pour over salad.

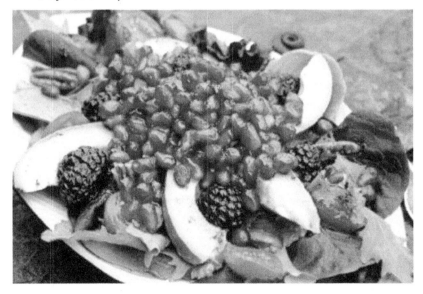

Superfoods Salad

Allergies: SF, GF

Typical superfoods salad should have:

1 part leafy greens - kale, spinach, dandelion and optional cilantro

1 part veggies -carrots, tomato, peppers, beets, broccoli, celery, and some pungent veggies - shallots, ginger or garlic

1 part fruits - pomegranates, avocado, blackberries, blueberries, sliced apple, grapefruit, raspberries, orange

1/2 part of nuts & seeds - almond, walnuts, chia, flax meal, sunflower seeds, pumpkin seeds

1 part protein - low-fat feta, yogurt, 2 boiled eggs or tuna

1 part cooked quinoa (optional)

Make your own mix and use different ingredient every time

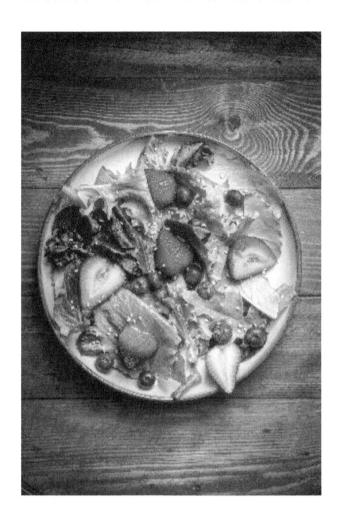

Apple Coleslaw

Serves 1-2

Ingredients - Allergies: SF, GF, DF, EF, V, NF

- 1 cup chopped cabbage (various color)
- 1 tart apple chopped
- 1 celery, chopped
- 1 red pepper chopped
- 5 tsp. olive oil or avocado oil
- juice of 1 lemon
- 2 Tbs raw honey (optional)
- dash sea salt

Instructions

Toss the cabbage, apple, celery, and pepper together in a large bowl. In a smaller bowl, whisk remaining ingredients. Drizzle over coleslaw and toss to coat.

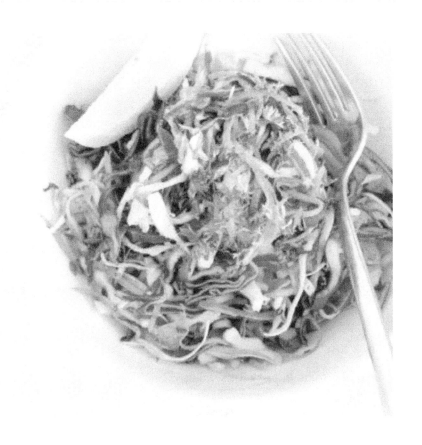

Appetizers

Hummus

Ingredients - Allergies: SF, GF, DF, EF, V, NF

- 2 cups cooked chickpeas (garbanzo beans)
- 1/4 cup (59 ml) fresh lemon juice, about 1 large lemon
- 1/4 cup (59 ml) tahini
- Half of a large garlic clove, minced
- 2 tbsp. olive oil or cumin oil, plus more for serving
- 1/2 to 1 tsp. salt
- 1/2 tsp. ground cumin
- 2 to 3 tbsp. water
- Dash of ground paprika for serving

Instructions

Combine tahini and lemon juice and blend for 1 minute. Add the olive oil, minced garlic, cumin and the salt to tahini and lemon mixture. Process for 30 seconds, scrape sides and then process 30 seconds more.

Add half of the chickpeas to the food processor and process for 1 minute. Scrape sides, add remaining chickpeas and process for 1 to 2 minutes.

Transfer the hummus into a bowl then drizzle about 1 tbsp. of olive oil over the top and sprinkle with paprika.

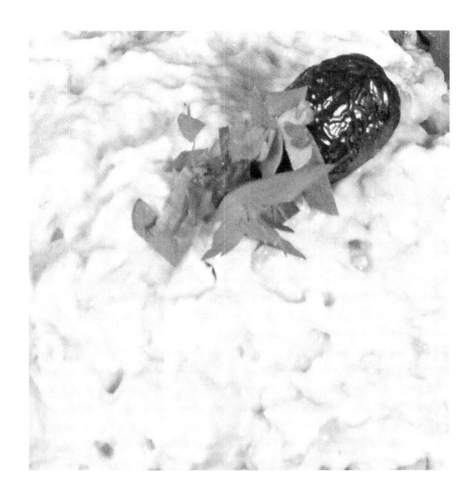

Guacamole

Ingredients - Allergies: SF, GF, DF, EF, V, NF

- 4 ripe avocados

- 3 tbsp. freshly squeezed lemon juice (1 lemon)

- 1/2 cup diced onion

- 1 large garlic clove, minced

- 1 tsp. salt

- 1 medium tomato, seeded, and small-diced

Instructions

Cut the avocados in half, remove the pits, and scoop the flesh out. Immediately add the lemon juice, hot pepper sauce, garlic, onion, salt, and pepper and toss well. Dice avocados. Add the tomatoes. Mix well and taste for salt and pepper.

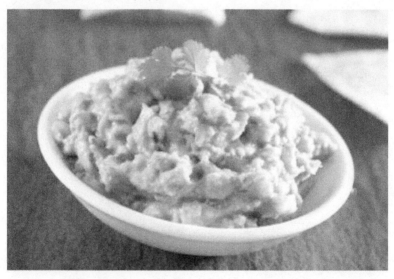

Baba Ghanoush

Ingredients - Allergies: SF, GF, DF, EF, V, NF

- 1 large eggplant
- 1/4 cup tahini, plus more as needed
- 3 garlic cloves, minced
- 1/4 cup fresh lemon juice, plus more as needed
- 1 pinch ground cumin
- salt, to taste
- 1 tbsp. extra-virgin olive oil or avocado oil
- 1 tbsp. chopped flat-leaf parsley
- 1/4 cup brine-cured black olives, such as Kalamata

Instructions:

Grill eggplant for 10 to 15 minutes. Heat the oven (375 F).

Put the eggplant to a baking sheet and bake 15-20 minutes or until very soft. Remove from the oven, let cool, and peel off and discard the skin. Put the eggplant flesh in a bowl. Using a fork, mash the eggplant to a paste.

Add the 1/4 cup tahini, garlic, cumin, 1/4 cup lemon juice and mix well. Season with salt to taste. Transfer the mixture to a serving bowl and spread with the back of a spoon to form a shallow well. Drizzle the olive oil over the top and sprinkle with the parsley.

Serve at room temperature.

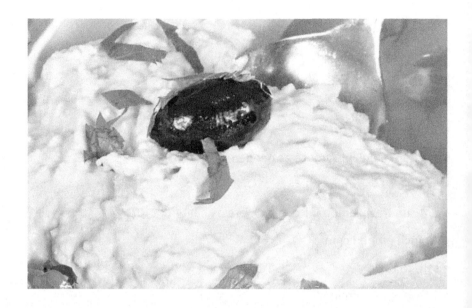

Tapenade

Ingredients - Allergies: SF, GF, DF, EF, V, NF

- 1/2 pound pitted mixed olives
- 2 anchovy fillets, rinsed
- 1 small clove garlic, minced
- 2 tbsp. capers
- 2 to 3 fresh basil leaves
- 1 tbsp. freshly squeezed lemon juice
- 2 tbsp. extra-virgin olive oil or cumin oil

Instructions

Rinse the olives in cool water. Place all ingredients in the bowl of a food processor. Process to combine, until it becomes a coarse paste. Transfer to a bowl and serve

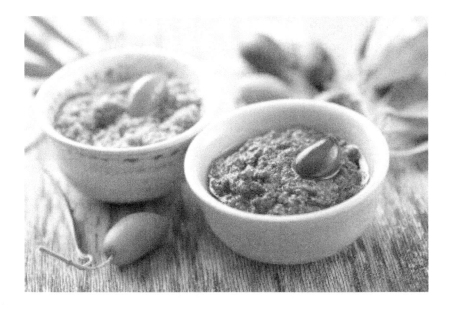

Red Pepper Dip

Ingredients - Allergies: SF, GF, EF, NF

- 1 pound red peppers

- 1 cup farmers' cheese

- 1/4 cup virgin <u>olive</u> oil or <u>avocado</u> oil

- 1 tbsp minced garlic

- Lemon juice, salt, basil, oregano, red pepper flakes to taste.

Instructions

Roast the peppers. Cover them and cool for about 15 minutes. Peel the peppers and remove the seeds and stems. Chop the peppers.

Transfer the peppers and garlic to a food processor and process until smooth. Add the farmers' cheese and garlic and process until smooth. With the machine running, add olive oil and lemon juice. Add the basil, oregano, red pepper flakes, and 1/4 tsp. salt, and process until smooth. Adjust the seasoning, to taste. Pour to a bowl. Refrigerate.

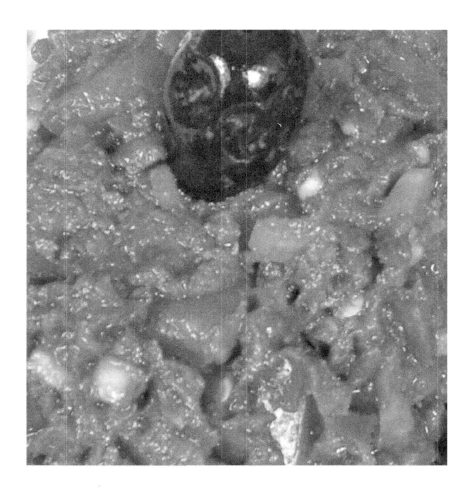

Eggplant and Yogurt

Instructions - Allergies: SF, GF, EF, NF

Mix 1 pound chopped eggplant, 3 unpeeled shallots and 3 unpeeled garlic cloves with 1/4 cup olive oil, salt and pepper on a baking sheet. Roast at 400 degrees for half an hour. Cool and squeeze the shallots and garlic from their skins and chop. Mix with the eggplant, almond, 1/2 cup plain yogurt, dill and salt and pepper.

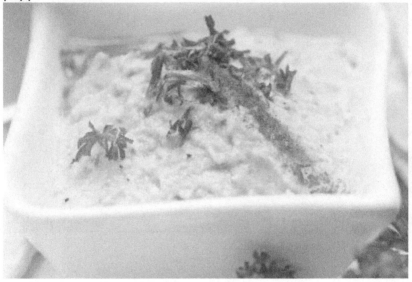

Caponata

Serves 3-4

Ingredients - Allergies: SF, GF, DF

- coconut oil
- 2 large eggplants, cut into large chunks
- 1 tsp. dried oregano
- Sea salt
- 1 small onion, peeled and finely chopped
- 2 cloves garlic, peeled and finely sliced
- 1 small bunch fresh flat-leaf parsley, leaves picked and stalks finely chopped
- 2 tbsp. salted capers, rinsed, soaked and drained
- 1 handful green olives, stones removed
- 2-3 tbsp. lemon juice
- 5 large ripe tomatoes, roughly chopped
- coconut oil
- 2 tbsp. slivered almonds, lightly toasted, optional

Instructions

Heat coconut oil in a pan and add eggplant, oregano and salt. Cook on a high heat for around 4 or 5 minutes. Add the onion, garlic and parsley stalks and continue cooking for another few minutes. Add drained capers and the olives and lemon juice. When all the juice has evaporated, add the tomatoes and simmer until tender.

Season with salt and olive oil to taste before serving. Sprinkle with almonds.

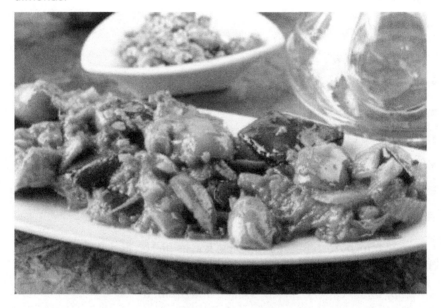

Soups

Cream of Broccoli Soup
Serves 4

Ingredients - Allergies: SF, GF, EF, NF

- 1 1/2 pounds broccoli, fresh
- 2 cups water
- 3/4 tsp. salt, pepper to taste
- 1/2 cup tapioca flour, mixed with 1 cup cold water
- 1/2 cup coconut cream

- 1/2 cup low-fat farmers cheese

Steam or boil broccoli until it gets tender.
Put 2 cups water and coconut cream in top of double boiler.
Add salt, cheese and pepper. Heat until cheese gets melted.
Add broccoli. Mix water and tapioca flour in a small bowl.
Stir tapioca mixture into cheese mixture in double boiler and heat until soup thickens.

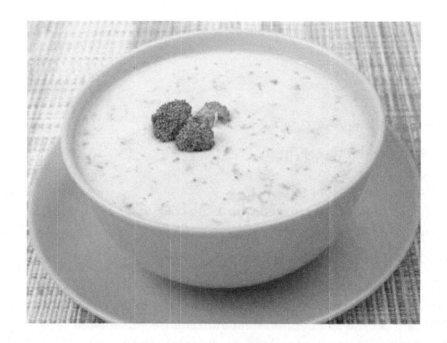

Lentil Soup

Serves 4-6

Ingredients - Allergies: SF, GF, DF, EF, NF
• 2 tbsp. olive oil or avocado oil
• 1 cup finely chopped onion
• 1/2 cup chopped carrot
• 1/2 cup chopped celery
• 2 teaspoons salt
• 1 pound lentils
• 1 cup chopped tomatoes
• 2 quarts chicken or vegetable broth
• 1/2 tsp. ground coriander & toasted cumin

Instructions

Place the olive oil into a large Dutch oven. Set over medium heat. Once hot, add the celery, onion, carrot and salt and do until the onions are translucent. Add the lentils, tomatoes, cumin, broth and coriander and stir to combine. Increase the heat and bring just to a boil. Reduce the heat, cover and simmer at a low until the lentils are tender (approx. 35 to 40 minutes). Puree with a bender to your preferred consistency (optional). Serve immediately.

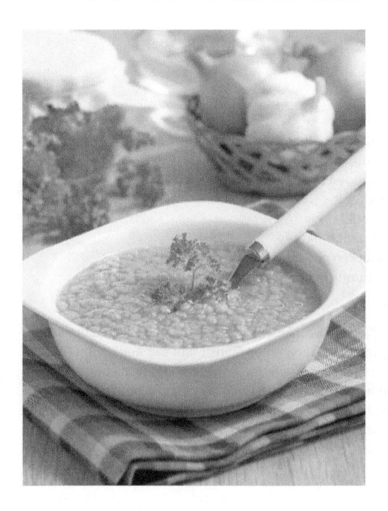

Cold Cucumber Avocado Soup
Serves 2-3

Ingredients - Allergies: SF, GF, EF, NF
• 1 cucumber peeled, seeded and cut into 2-inch chunks
• 1 avocado, peeled
• 2 chopped scallions
• 1 cup chicken broth
• 3/4 cup Greek low-fat yogurt
• 2 tbsp. lemon juice
• 1/2 tsp. ground pepper, or to taste
Garnish:
• Chopped chives, dill, mint, scallions or cucumber
Instructions
Combine the cucumber, avocado and scallions in a blender. Pulse until chopped.
Add yogurt, broth and lemon juice and continue until smooth.
Season with pepper and salt to taste and chill for 4 hours.
Taste for seasoning and garnish.

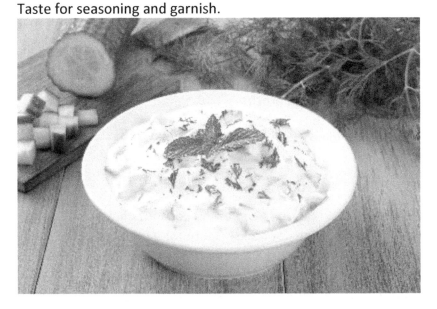

Bouillabaisse

Serves 6.

Ingredients - Allergies: SF, GF, DF, EF, NF

- 3 pounds of 3 different kinds of fish fillets
- 1/2 cup coconut oil
- 1-2 pounds of Oysters, clams, or mussels
- 1 cup cooked shrimp, crab, or lobster meat, or rock lobster tails
- 1 cup thinly sliced onions
- 4 Shallots or the white parts of 2 or 3 leeks, thinly sliced
- 2 cloves garlic, crushed
- 1 large tomato, chopped
- 1 sweet red pepper, chopped
- 4 stalks celery, thinly sliced
- 2-inch slice of fennel or 1 tsp. of fennel seed
- 3 sprigs fresh thyme or 3/4 tsp. dried thyme
- 1 bay leaf
- 2-3 whole cloves
- Zest of half an orange
- 1/2 tsp. saffron
- 2 teaspoons salt
- 1 cup clam juice or fish broth
- 2 Tbps lemon juice
- 2/3 cup white wine

Instructions

In a large saucepan heat 1/4 cup of the coconut oil. When it is hot, add onions and shallots (or leeks). Sauté for a minute. Add crushed garlic, and sweet red pepper. Add celery, tomato, and fennel. Stir the vegetables until well coated. Add another 1/4 cup of coconut oil, bay leaf, thyme, cloves and the orange zest. Cook until the onion is golden. Cut fish fillets into 2-inch pieces. Add 2 cups of water and the pieces of fish to the vegetable mixture. Bring to a boil, then reduce heat and let it simmer, uncovered, for about 10 minutes. Add clams, oysters or mussels (optional) and crabmeat, shrimp or lobster tails, cut into pieces. Add salt, saffron and pepper. Add lemon juice, clam juice, and white wine. Bring to a simmer again and cook for 5 minutes longer.

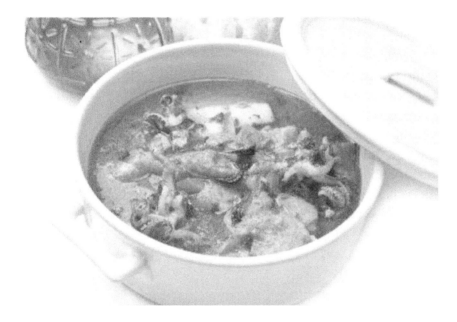

Gaspacho

Serves 4

Ingredients - Allergies: SF, GF, DF, EF, V, NF

- 1/2 cup of <u>flax</u> seeds meal
- 1kg tomatoes, diced
- 1 red pepper and 1 green pepper, diced
- 1 cucumber, peeled and diced
- 2 cloves of garlic, peeled and crushed
- 150ml extra virgin <u>olive</u> oil or <u>avocado</u> oil
- 2tbsp lemon juice
- Salt, to taste

Instructions

Mix the peppers, tomatoes and cucumber with the crushed garlic and olive oil in the bowl of a blender. Add flax meal to the mixture. Blend until smooth. Add salt and lemon juice to taste and stir well. Refrigerate until well chilled. Serve with black olives, hard-boiled egg, cilantro, mint or parsley.

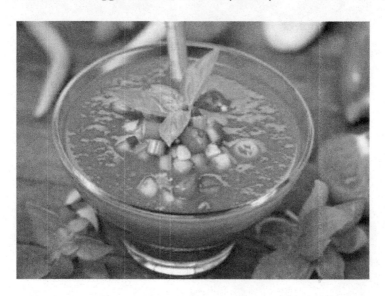

Italian Beef Soup
Serves 6

Ingredients - Allergies: SF, GF, DF, EF, NF

- 1 pound minced beef
- 1 clove garlic, minced
- 2 cups beef broth
- few large tomatoes
- 1 cup sliced carrots
- 2 cups cooked beans
- 2 small zucchini, cubed
- 2 cups spinach - rinsed and torn
- 1/4 tsp. salt

Brown beef with garlic in a stockpot. Stir in broth, carrots and tomatoes. Season with salt and pepper. Reduce heat, cover, and simmer for 15 minutes.
Stir in beans with liquid and zucchini. Cover, and simmer until zucchini is tender. Remove from heat, add spinach and cover. Serve after 5 minutes.

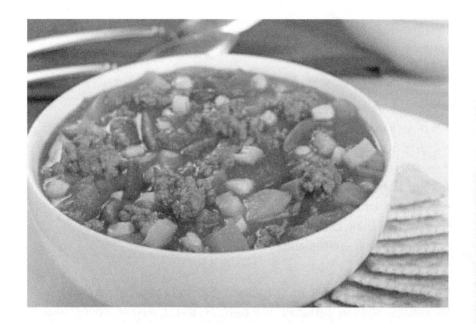

Creamy roasted mushroom

Serves 4

Ingredients - Allergies: SF, GF, DF, EF, V, NF

- 1 pound Portobello mushrooms, cut into 1inch pieces
- 1/2 pound shiitake mushrooms, stemmed
- 6 tbsp. olive oil or avocado oil
- 2 cups vegetable broth
- 1 1/2 tbsp. coconut oil
- 1 onion, chopped
- 3 garlic cloves, minced
- 3 tbsp. arrowroot flour
- 1 cup coconut cream
- 3/4 tsp. chopped thyme

Instructions

Heat oven to 400°F. Line one large baking sheets with foil. Spread mushrooms and drizzle some olive oil on them. Season with salt and pepper and toss. Cover with foil and bake them for half an hour. Uncover and continue baking 15 minutes more. Cool slightly. Mix one half of the mushrooms with one can of broth in a blender. Set aside.

Melt coconut oil in a large pot over high heat. Add onion and garlic and sauté until onion is translucent. Add flour and stir 2 minutes. Add cream, broth, and thyme. Stir in remaining cooked mushrooms and mushroom puree. Simmer over low heat until thickened (approx. 10 minutes). Season to taste with salt and pepper.

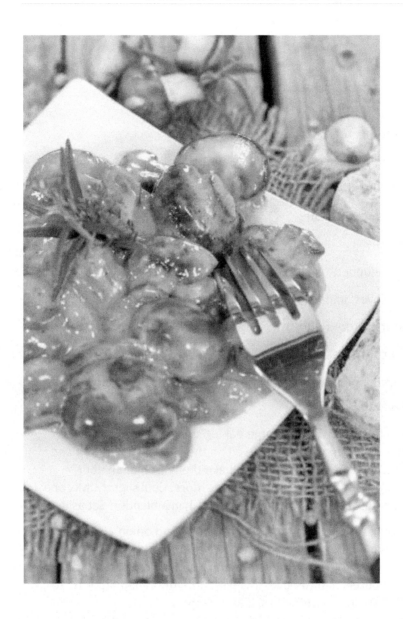

Black Bean Soup

Serves 6-8

Ingredients - Allergies: SF, GF, DF, EF, NF

- 1/4 cup coconut oil
- 1/4 cup Onion, Diced
- 1/4 cup Carrots, Diced
- 1/4 cup Green Bell Pepper, Diced
- 1 cup beef broth
- 3 pounds cooked Black Beans
- 1 tbsp. lemon juice
- 2 teaspoons Garlic
- 2 teaspoons Salt
- 2 teaspoons Chili Powder
- 8 oz. pork
- 1 tbsp. tapioca flour
- 2 tbsp. Water

Instructions

Place coconut oil, onion, carrot, and bell pepper in a stock pot. Cook the veggies until tender. Bring broth to a boil. Add cooked beans, broth and the remaining ingredients (except tapioca flour and 2 tbsp. water) to the vegetables. Bring that mixture to a simmer and cook approximately 15 minutes. Puree 1 quart of the soup in a blender and put back into the pot. Combine the tapioca flour and 2 tbsp. water in a separate bowl. Add the tapioca flour mixture to the bean soup and bring to a boil for 1 minute.

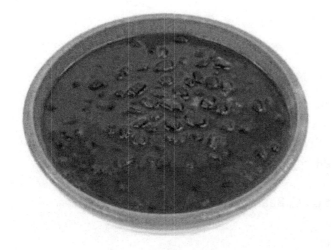

Squash soup
Serves 4-6

Ingredients - Allergies: SF, GF, DF, EF, V, NF

• 1 Squash

• 1 carrot, chopped

• 1 onion (diced)

• 3/4 – 1 cup coconut milk

• 1/4 – 1/2 cup water

• olive oil or avocado oil

• Salt

• Pepper

• Cinnamon

• Turmeric

Instructions

Cut the squash and spoon out the seeds. Cut it into large pieces and place on a baking sheet. Sprinkle with salt, olive oil, and pepper and bake at 375 degrees F until soft (approx. 1 hour). Let cool.

In the meantime, sauté the onions in olive oil (put it in a soup pot). Add the carrots. Add 3/4 cup coconut milk and 1/4 cup water after few minutes and let simmer. Scoop the squash out of its skin. Add it to the soup pot. Stir to combine the ingredients and let simmer a few minutes. Add more milk or water if needed. Season to taste with the salt, pepper and spices. Blend until smooth and creamy.

Sprinkle it with toasted pumpkin seeds.

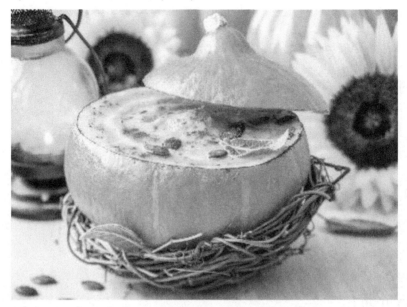

Avgolemono – Greek lemon chicken soup

Serves 4

Ingredients - Allergies: SF, GF, DF, EF, NF

- 4 cups chicken broth
- 1/4 cup uncooked quinoa
- salt and pepper
- 3 eggs
- 3 tbsp. lemon juice
- Handful fresh dill (chopped)
- shredded roasted chicken (optional)

Bring the broth to a boil in a saucepan. Add the quinoa and cook until tender. Season with the salt and pepper. Reduce heat to low and let simmer. In a separate bowl, whisk lemon juice and the eggs until smooth. Add about 1 cup of the hot broth into the egg/lemon mixture and whisk to combine.

Add the mixture back to the saucepan. Stir until the soup becomes opaque and thickens. Add dill, salt and pepper to taste and chicken if you have it, and serve.

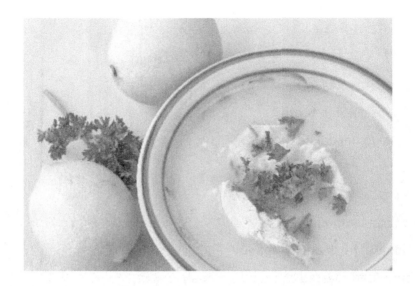

Egg-Drop Soup

Serves 4-6

Ingredients - Allergies: SF, GF, DF, NF

- 1 1/2 quarts chicken broth
- 2 tbsps. Tapioca flour, mixed in 1/4 cup cold water
- 2 eggs, slightly beaten with a fork
- 2 scallions, chopped, including green ends

Instructions

Bring broth to a boil. Slowly pour in the tapioca flour mixture while stirring the broth. The broth should thicken. Reduce heat and let it simmer. Mix in the eggs very slowly while stirring. As soon as the last drop of egg is in, turn off the heat. Serve with chopped scallions on top.

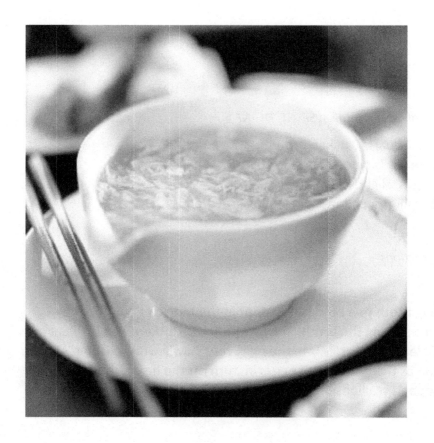

Creamy Tomato Basil Soup

Serves 6

Ingredients - Allergies: SF, GF, DF, EF, V, NF

- 4 tomatoes - peeled, seeded and diced
- 4 cups tomato juice*
- 14 leaves fresh basil
- 1 cup coconut cream
- salt to taste

Instructions

Combine tomatoes and tomato juice in stock pot. Simmer 30 minutes. Puree mixture with basil leaves in a processor. Put back in a stock pot and add coconut cream. Add salt and pepper to taste.

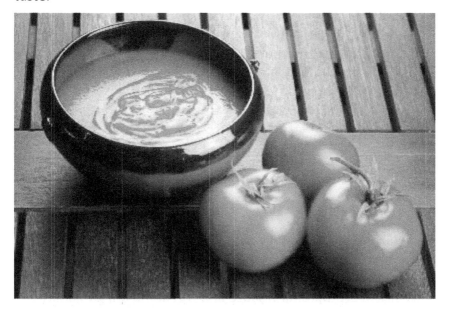

Minestrone

Serves 8-10

Ingredients - Allergies: SF, GF, DF, EF, NF

- 3 tbsp. coconut oil
- 3 cloves garlic, chopped
- 2 onions, chopped
- 2 cups chopped celery
- 5 carrots, sliced
- 2 cups chicken broth
- 2 cups water
- 4 cups tomato sauce
- 1/2 oz. red wine (optional)
- 1 cup cooked kidney beans
- 2 cups green beans
- 2 cups baby spinach, rinsed
- 3 zucchinis, quartered and sliced
- 1 tbsp. chopped oregano
- 2 tbsp. chopped basil
- salt and pepper to taste
- 1 tbsp. olive oil or cumin oil

Instructions

Heat coconut oil over medium heat in a stock pot, and sauté garlic for few minutes. Add onion and sauté for few more minutes. Add celery and carrots and sauté for 2 minutes.

Add chicken broth, tomato sauce and water and bring to boil, stirring frequently. Add red wine at this point. Reduce heat to low and add kidney beans, zucchini, green beans, spinach leaves, oregano, basil, salt and pepper. Simmer for 30 to 40 minutes.

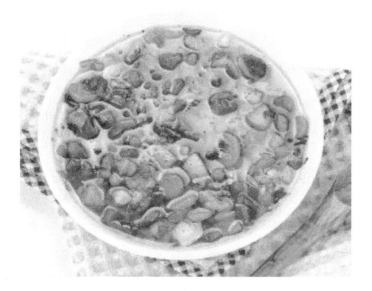

Grilled Meats & Salad

Chicken and Large Fiber Loaded Salad with Italian Dressing

Serves 1 - Allergies: SF, GF, EF, NF

• 6oz. of Chicken (or turkey), skinless, boneless grilled or prepared in the skillet.

• Large mixed spinach and lettuce salad with Italian Dressing and half a tsp of mustard. Salad can be as large as you want, but use half a cup of the dressing.

• Salad with Yogurt Dressing would have 80 calories more (330 calories total)

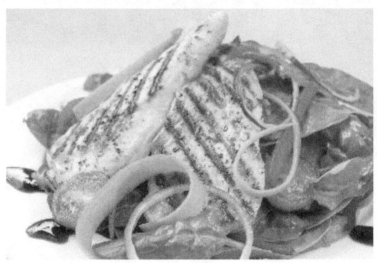

Nutrition Facts

Serving Size 247 g

Amount Per Serving

Calories 252   Calories from Fat 122

% **Daily Value***

Total Fat 13.6g	**21%**
Saturated Fat 2.0g	**10%**
Trans Fat 0.0g	
Cholesterol 63mg	**21%**
Sodium 99mg	**4%**
Potassium 831mg	**24%**
Total Carbohydrates 5.1g	**2%**
Dietary Fiber 2.4g	**10%**
Sugars 2.4g	
Protein 29.3g	

Vitamin A 60%	Vitamin C 57%
Calcium 11%	Iron 11%

Nutrition Grade B+

* Based on a 2000 calorie diet

Salmon with Large Fiber Loaded Salad with Italian Dressing

Serves 1 - Allergies: SF, GF, DF, EF, NF

• 4oz. of Salmon grilled or prepared in the skillet.

• Large mixed spinach and lettuce salad with "Italian Dressing" and some thyme sprinkled on top of it. Salad can be as large as you want, but use the prescribed amount of the dressing.

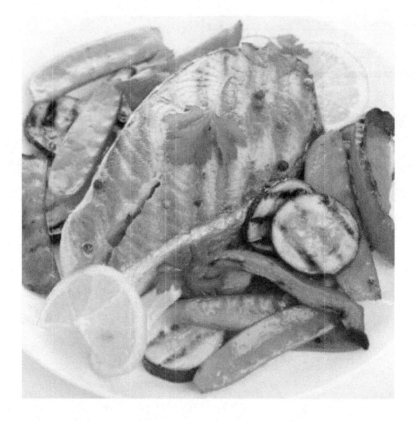

Herb Crusted Salmon

Serves 1 - Allergies: SF, GF, DF, EF, NF

Rub some tarragon, chives and parsley over 4 oz. salmon and add some salt and pepper. Heat the pan with 1 tsp of coconut oil to medium high and place the salmon, skin-side up in the pan. Cook until golden brown on 1 side, about 4 minutes. Turn the fish over and cook until it feels firm to the touch. Salmon is done when it flakes easily with a fork. Serve with a lemon wedge.

• Large mixed spinach and lettuce salad with "Italian Dressing" and some thyme sprinkled on top of it. Salad can be as large as you want, but use the prescribed amount of the dressing.

Nutrition Facts

Serving Size 247 g

Amount Per Serving

Calories 252	Calories from Fat 122
	% Daily Value*
Total Fat 13.6g	**21%**
Saturated Fat 2.0g	**10%**
Trans Fat 0.0g	
Cholesterol 63mg	**21%**
Sodium 99mg	**4%**
Potassium 831mg	**24%**
Total Carbohydrates 5.1g	**2%**
Dietary Fiber 2.4g	**10%**
Sugars 2.4g	
Protein 29.3g	

Vitamin A 60%	•	Vitamin C 57%
Calcium 11%	•	Iron 11%

Nutrition Grade B+

* Based on a 2000 calorie diet

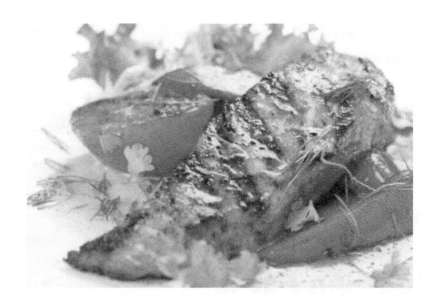

Ground Beef Patty with Large Fiber Loaded Salad with Yogurt Dressing

Serves 1 - Allergies: SF, GF, EF, NF

• 5oz. lean ground beef patty grilled or prepared in the skillet.

• Large mixed spinach and shredded cabbage salad with Yogurt Dressing. Salad can be as large as you want, but use half a cup of a dressing.

Nutrition Facts

Serving Size 247 g

Amount Per Serving

Calories 328	Calories from Fat 123

	% Daily Value*
Total Fat 13.7g	**21%**
Saturated Fat 4.0g	**20%**
Cholesterol 127mg	**42%**
Sodium 130mg	**5%**
Potassium 857mg	**24%**
Total Carbohydrates 5.1g	**2%**
Dietary Fiber 2.4g	**10%**
Sugars 2.4g	
Protein 44.8g	

Vitamin A 58%	•	Vitamin C 57%
Calcium 6%	•	Iron 155%

Nutrition Grade A

* Based on a 2000 calorie diet

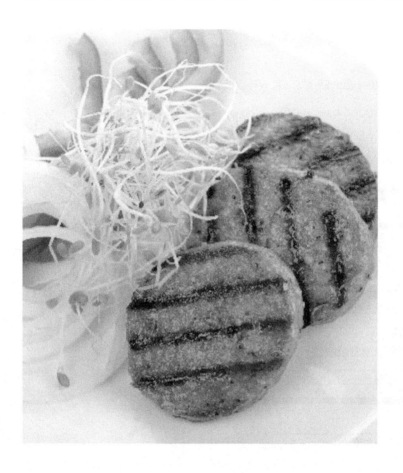

Lean Pork with Fiber Loaded Salad with Yogurt Dressing

Serves 1 - Allergies: SF, GF, EF, NF

• 5oz. of lean Pork Tenderloin grilled or prepared in the skillet.

• Large mixed spinach and shredded cabbage salad with Yogurt Dressing and half a tsp of mustard. Salad can be as large as you want, but use half a cup of the dressing.

Nutrition Facts

Serving Size 275 g

Amount Per Serving

Calories 231   Calories from Fat 71

	% Daily Value*
Total Fat 7.9g	12%
Saturated Fat 1.5g	7%
Trans Fat 0.0g	
Cholesterol 99mg	33%
Sodium 249mg	10%
Potassium 818mg	23%
Total Carbohydrates 5.1g	2%
Dietary Fiber 2.4g	10%
Sugars 2.4g	
Protein 33.6g	

Vitamin A 58%	•	Vitamin C 57%
Calcium 6%	•	Iron 15%

Nutrition Grade B-

* Based on a 2000 calorie diet

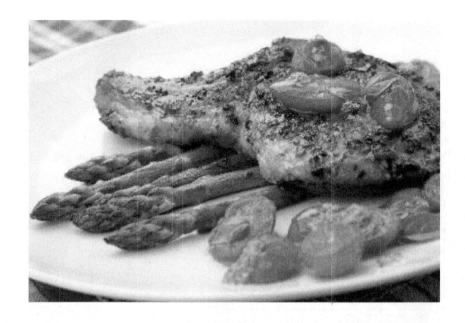

Caribbean Chicken salad

Serves 2

Ingredients - Allergies: SF, GF, DF, EF, NF

2 boneless skinless chicken breasts

Marinade

1/2 cup fish sauce

2 tomatoes (seeded and chopped)

1/2 cup chopped onion

2 tsps. jalapeno chilies (minced)

2 tsps. chopped cilantro fresh

Raw honey Lime Dressing:

1/4 cup mustard

1/4 cup raw honey

1 tbsp coconut oil

1 1/2 tbsps. lemon juice

1 1/2 tsps. lime juice

3/4 lb mixed greens

Instructions

Blend all the marinade ingredients in a small bowl with a hand blender. Cover and chill. Marinate the chicken for at least two hours in the fridge. Grill the chicken for few minutes per side or until done.

Serve the greens into 2 large salad bowls.
Slice the chicken into thin strips. Divide among bowls.
Pour the dressing aside and serve with the salads.

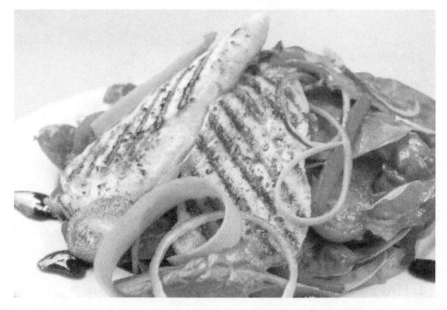

Tuna with Large Fiber Loaded Salad with Italian Dressing

Serves 1 - Allergies: SF, GF, DF, EF, NF

• 6 oz. can of Tuna, drained.

• Large mixed spinach and green onion salad with Italian Dressing and half a tsp of mustard. Salad can be as large as you want, but use only the prescribed amount of dressing. You may use fish sauce instead of salt.

Nutrition Facts

Serving Size 155 g

Amount Per Serving

Calories 275   Calories from Fat 134

	% Daily Value*
Total Fat 14.8g	**23%**
Saturated Fat 2.7g	**13%**
Cholesterol 37mg	**12%**
Sodium 83mg	**3%**
Potassium 574mg	**16%**
Total Carbohydrates 1.7g	**1%**
Dietary Fiber 0.9g	**4%**
Protein 32.8g	

Vitamin A 58%	•	Vitamin C 14%
Calcium 4%	•	Iron 10%

Nutrition Grade B+

* Based on a 2000 calorie diet

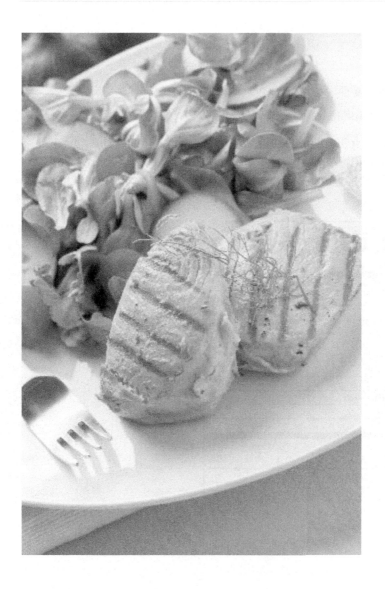

Stews, Chilies and Curries

Stuffed Peppers with beans
Serves 2

Ingredients - Allergies: SF, GF, DF, EF, V, NF

2 large red or green bell peppers
1 cup stewed tomatoes
1/3 cup brown rice
2 tbsp. hot water
2 green onions
8 ounces cooked black beans
1/4 tsp. crushed red pepper flakes

Instructions

Discard seeds and membrane from peppers. Place cut-side down and cover. Bake at 375F for 15 minutes.
While the peppers are cooking, cook tomatoes, rice and water for 15 minutes. In the meantime, thinly slice green onions.
Stir beans, green onions, and pepper flakes into tomato mixture. Cook for 10 minutes more. Drain peppers. Turn cut-side up. Spoon beans mixture evenly into peppers and bake in the oven for 5-10 minutes.

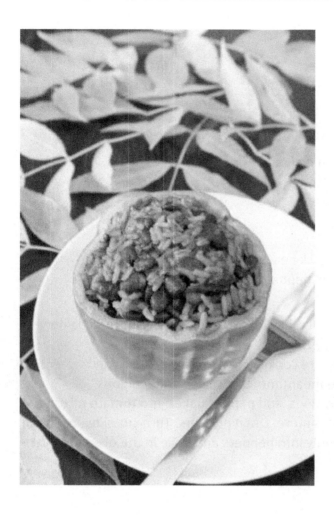

Vegetarian Chili

Serves 4-6

Ingredients - Allergies: SF, GF, DF, EF, V, NF

1 tbsp. coconut oil
1 cup chopped onions
3/4 cup chopped carrots
3 cloves garlic, minced
1 cup chopped green bell pepper
1 cup chopped red bell pepper
3/4 cup chopped celery
1 tbsp. chili powder
1-1/2 cups chopped mushrooms
3 cups chopped tomatoes
2 cups cooked kidney beans
1 tbsp. ground cumin
1-1/2 teaspoons oregano
1-1/2 teaspoons crushed basil leaves

Instructions

Heat coconut oil in a large saucepan and add onions, carrots and garlic; sauté until tender. Stir in green pepper, red pepper, celery and chili powder.
Cook, stirring often, until vegetables are tender, about 6 minutes. To the vegetables add mushrooms; cook 4 minutes. Stir in tomatoes, kidney beans, corn, cumin, oregano and basil. Bring to a boil. Reduce heat to medium. Cover and simmer for 20 minutes, stirring occasionally.

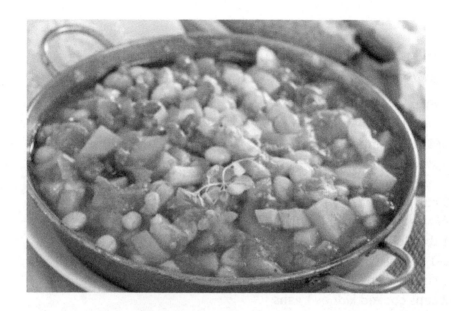

Lentil Stew

Recipe is for 4 servings, but you might want to adjust to 2 servings (eat one, freeze one)

Ingredients - Allergies: SF, GF, DF, EF, NF

- 1 cup dry lentils

- 3 1/2 cups chicken broth

- few tomatoes

- 1 medium potato chopped + 1/2 cup chopped carrot

- 1/2 cup chopped onion + 1/2 cup chopped celery (optional)

- few sprigs of parsley and basil + 1 garlic clove (minced)

- 1 pound of cubed lean pork or beef + pepper to taste

Nutrition Facts

Serving Size 456 g

Amount Per Serving

Calories 453	Calories from Fat 79

	% Daily Value*
Total Fat 8.8g	**14%**
Saturated Fat 3.0g	**15%**
Trans Fat 0.0g	
Cholesterol 101mg	**34%**
Sodium 684mg	**29%**
Potassium 1394mg	**40%**
Total Carbohydrates 39.4g	**13%**
Dietary Fiber 16.8g	**67%**
Sugars 4.8g	
Protein 51.7g	

Vitamin A 13%	•	Vitamin C 28%
Calcium 5%	•	Iron 148%

Nutrition Grade A

* Based on a 2000 calorie diet

You can eat a salad of your choice with this stew.

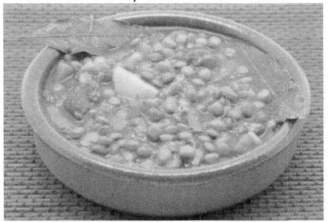

White Chicken Chili

Serves: 5

Ingredients - Allergies: SF, GF, DF, EF, NF

- 4 large boneless, skinless chicken breasts
- 2 green bell peppers
- 1 large yellow onion
- 1 jalapeno
- 1/2 cup diced green chilies (optional)
- 1/2 cup of spring onions
- 1.5 tbsp. coconut oil
- 3 cups cooked white beans
- 3.5 cups chicken or vegetable broth
- 1 tsp. ground cumin
- 1/4 tsp. cayenne pepper
- salt to taste

Instructions

Bring a pot of water to boil. Add the chicken breasts and cook until cooked through. Drain water and allow chicken to cool. When cool, shred and set aside.

Dice the bell peppers, jalapeno and onion. Melt the coconut oil in a pot over high heat. Add the peppers and onions and sauté until soft, approx. 8-10 minutes.

Add the broth, beans, chicken and spices to the pot. Stir and bring to a low boil. Cover and simmer for 25-30 minutes.

Simmer for 10 more minutes and stir occasionally. Remove from heat. Let stand for 10 minutes to thicken. Top with cilantro.

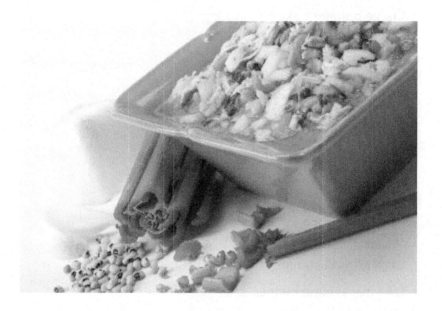

Ratatouille

Serves 4-6

Ingredients - Allergies: SF, GF, DF, EF, V, NF

- 2 large eggplants
- 3 medium zucchinis
- 2 medium onions
- 2 red or green peppers
- 4 large tomatoes
- 2 cloves garlic, crushed
- 4 tbsp. coconut oil
- 1 tbsp. fresh basil
- Salt

Instructions

Cut eggplant and zucchini into 1 inch slices. Then cut each slice in half. Salt them and leave them for one hour. The salt will draw out the bitterness.

Chop peppers and onions. Skin the tomatoes by boiling them for few minutes. Then quarter them, take out the seeds and chop the flesh. Fry garlic and the onions in the coconut oil in a saucepan for a 10 minutes. Add the peppers. Dry the eggplant and zucchini and add them to the saucepan. Add the basil, salt and pepper. Stir and simmer for half an hour.

Add the tomato flesh, check the seasoning and cook for an additional 15 minutes with the lid off.

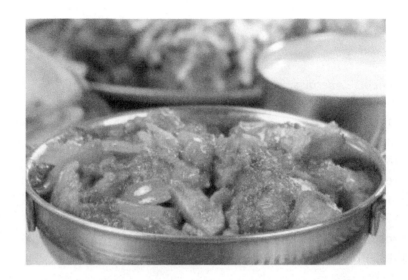

Barbecued Beef

Serves 8

Ingredients - Allergies: SF, GF, DF, EF, NF

- 1-1/2 cups tomato paste
- 1/4 cup lemon juice
- 2 tbsp. mustard
- 1/2 tsp. salt
- 1 chopped carrot
- 1/2 tsp. minced garlic
- 4 pounds boneless chuck roast

Instructions

In a large bowl, combine tomato paste, lemon juice and mustard. Stir in salt, pepper and garlic.

Place chuck roast and carrot in a slow cooker. Pour tomato mixture over chuck roast. Cover, and cook on low for 7 to 9 hours. Remove chuck roast from slow cooker, shred with a fork, and return to the slow cooker. Stir meat to evenly coat with sauce. Continue cooking approximately 1 hour.

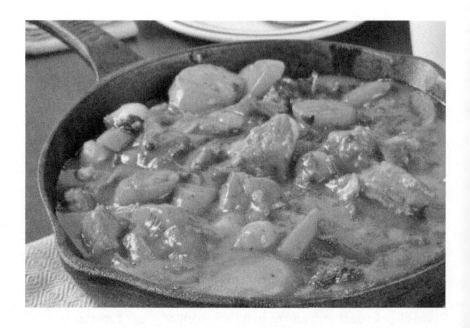

Beef Tenderloin with Roasted Shallots

Serves 4-6

Ingredients - Allergies: SF, GF, DF, EF

- 3/4 pound shallots, halved lengthwise and peeled
- 1-1/2 tbsp. olive oil or avocado oil
- salt and pepper to taste
- 3 cups beef broth
- 3/4 cup red wine
- 1-1/2 teaspoons tomato paste
- 2 pounds beef tenderloin roast, trimmed
- 1 tsp. dried thyme
- 3 tbsp. coconut oil
- 1 tbsp. almond flour

Instructions

Heat oven to 375 degrees F. Toss shallots with olive oil to coat in a baking pan and season with salt and pepper. Roast until shallots are tender, stirring occasionally, about half an hour.
Combine wine and beef broth in a sauce pan and bring to a boil. Cook over high heat. Volume should be reduced by half. Add in tomato paste. Set aside.
Pat beef dry and sprinkle with salt and thyme and pepper. Add beef to pan oiled with coconut oil. Brown on all sides over high heat.
Put pan back to the oven. Roast beef about half an hour for medium rare. Transfer beef to platter. Cover loosely with foil.
Place pan on stove top and add broth mixture. Bring to boil and stir to scrape up any browned bits. Transfer to a different saucepan, and bring to simmer. Mix 1 1/2 tbsp. coconut oil and

flour in small bowl and mix. Whisk into broth, and simmer until sauce thickens. Stir in roasted shallots. Season with salt and pepper.

Cut beef into 1/2 inch thick slices. Spoon some sauce over.

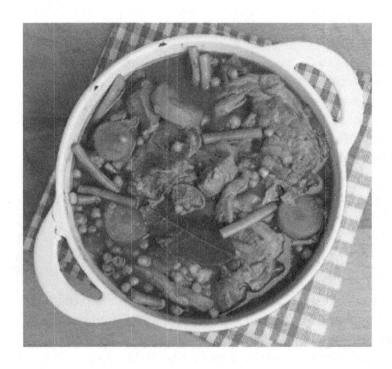

Superfoods Chili
Serves 6

Ingredients - Allergies: SF, GF, DF, EF, NF

- 2 tbsp. coconut oil
- 2 onions, chopped
- 3 cloves garlic, minced
- 1 pound ground beef
- 3/4 pound beef sirloin, cubed
- 2cups diced tomatoes
- 1 cup strong brewed coffee
- 1cup tomato paste
- 2 cups beef broth
- 1 tbsp. cumin seeds
- 1 tbsp. unsweetened cocoa powder
- 1 tsp. dried oregano
- 1 tsp. ground cayenne pepper
- 1 tsp. ground coriander
- 1 tsp. salt
- 6 cups cooked kidney beans
- 4 fresh hot chili peppers, chopped

Instructions

Heat oil in a saucepan over medium heat. Cook garlic, onions, sirloin and ground beef in oil until the meat is browned and the onions are translucent.
Mix in the diced tomatoes, coffee, tomato paste and beef broth. Season with oregano, cumin, cocoa powder, cayenne pepper, coriander and salt. Stir in hot chile peppers and 3 cups of the beans. Reduce heat to low, and simmer for two hours.

Stir in the 3 remaining cups of beans. Simmer for another 30 minutes.

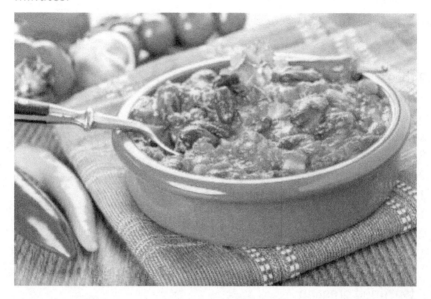

Glazed Meatloaf

Serves 4

Ingredients - Allergies: SF, GF, DF, NF

- 1/2 cup tomato paste
- 1/4 cup lemon juice, divided
- 1 tsp. mustard powder
- 2 pounds ground beef
- 1 cup flax seeds meal

- 1/4 cup chopped onion
- 1 egg, beaten

Instructions

Heat oven to 350 degrees F. Combine mustard, tomato paste, 1 tbsp. lemon juice in a small bowl.

Combine onion, ground beef, flax, egg and remaining lemon juice in a separate larger bowl. And add 1/3 of the tomato paste mixture from the smaller bowl. Mix all well and place in a loaf pan.

Bake at 350 degrees F for one hour. Drain any excess fat and coat with remaining tomato paste mixture. Bake for 10 more minutes.

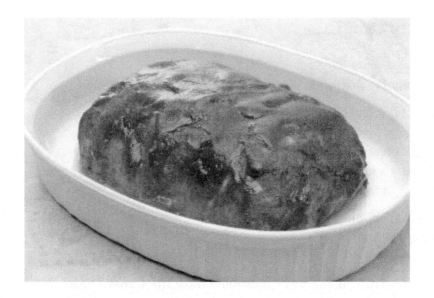

Eggplant Lasagna

Serves 4-6

Ingredients - Allergies: SF, GF, NF

- 2 large eggplants, peeled and sliced lengthwise into strips
- coconut oil
- salt and pepper

Meat Sauce

- 1 1/2 lbs ground sirloin or 1 1/2 lbs turkey breast
- 2 tbsp. coconut oil
- 2 onions, chopped
- 3 cloves chopped garlic
- 1 red pepper, chopped
- 1 (16 ounce) package sliced mushrooms
- 1 tbsp. of oregano, basil and thyme each
- 1 tsp. fennel seed (optional)
- salt and pepper
- 1 tsp. red pepper flakes (optional)
- 1 cup chopped spinach
- 2 cups tomato sauce
- 1 cup diced tomatoes

Cheese Mixture

- 2 cups low-fat farmers cheese
- 2 eggs
- 3 green onions, chopped

• 1 cup shredded low-fat mozzarella cheese (optional)

Instructions

Heat oven to 425 degrees.

Oil cookie sheet and arrange eggplant slice. Sprinkle with salt and pepper. Bake slices 5 minutes on each side. Lower oven temp to 375.

Brown onion, meat and garlic in coconut oil for 5 minutes. Add mushrooms and red pepper, and cook for 5 minutes. Add tomatoes, spinach and spices and simmer for 5-10 minutes.

Blend farmers' cheese, egg and onion mixture. Spread one third of meat sauce in bottom of a glass pan. Layer one half of eggplant slices and one half farmers' cheese. Repeat. Add last layer of sauce and then mozzarella on top.

Cover with foil. Bake at 375 degrees for one hour. Remove foil and bake until cheese is browned. Let it rest 10 minutes before serving.

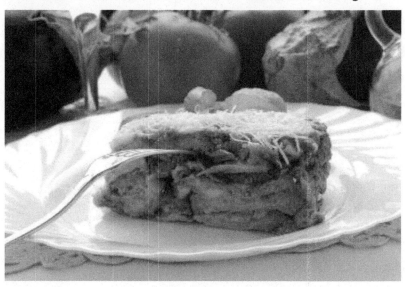

Stuffed Eggplant

Serves – one half of eggplant per person

Allergies: SF, GF, DF, EF, NF

Rinse the eggplants. Cut off a slice from one end. Make a wide slit and salt them. Deseed tomatoes. Chop them finely. Cut the onions in thin slices. Chop the garlic cloves. Place them in a frying pan with coconut oil. Add the tomatoes, salt parsley, cumin, pepper, hot peppers and ground beef. Sauté for 10 minutes.

Squeeze eggplants, so the bitter juice goes out. Fill the wide slit with the ground beef mix. Pour the remaining mix over. Heat the oven to 375F in the meantime. Place eggplants a baking pan. Sprinkle them with olive oil, lemon juice and 1 cup of water. Cover the pan with a foil.

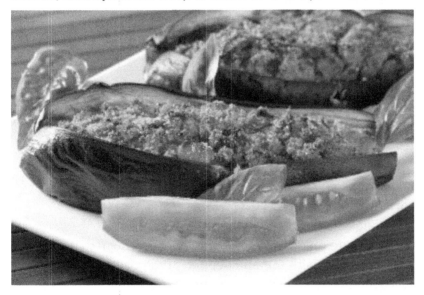

Stuffed Red Peppers with Beef

Serves 4-6

Ingredients - Allergies: SF, GF, DF, EF, NF

- 6 red bell peppers
- salt to taste
- 1 pound ground beef
- 1/3 cup chopped onion
- salt and pepper to taste
- 2 cups chopped tomatoes
- 1/2 cup uncooked brown rice or quinoa
- 1/2 cup water
- 2 cups tomato soup
- water as needed

Instructions

Bring a pot of salted water to a boil. Cut the tops off the peppers. Remove the seeds. Cook peppers in boiling water for 5 minutes and drain.
Sprinkle salt inside each pepper, and set aside.
In a skillet, sauté onions and beef until beef is browned. Drain off excess fat. Season with salt and pepper. Stir in rice, tomatoes and 1/2 cup water. Cover, and simmer until rice is tender. Remove from heat. Stir in the cheese.
Heat the oven to 350 degrees F. Stuff each pepper with the rice and beef mixture. Place peppers open side up in a baking dish. Combine tomato soup with just enough water to make the soup a gravy consistency in a separate bowl. Pour over the peppers.
Bake covered for 25 to 35 minutes.

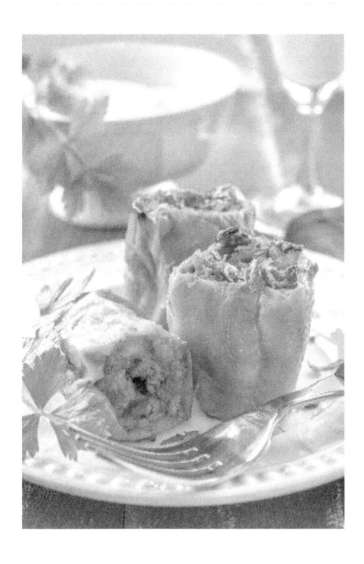

Superfoods Goulash

Serves 4-6

Ingredients - Allergies: SF, GF, DF, EF, NF

- 3 cups cauliflower
- 1 pound ground beef
- 1 medium onion, chopped
- salt to taste
- garlic to taste
- 2 cups cooked kidney beans
- 1 cup tomato paste

Brown the ground beef and onion in a skillet, over medium heat. Drain off the fat. Add garlic, salt and pepper to taste.
Stir in the cauliflower, kidney beans and tomato paste. Cook until cauliflower is done.

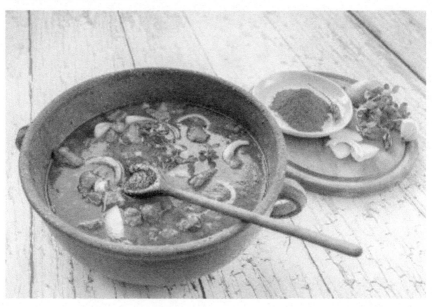

Frijoles Charros

Serves 4-6

Ingredients - Allergies: SF, GF, DF, EF, NF

- 1 pound dry pinto beans
- 5 cloves garlic, chopped
- 1 tsp. salt
- 1/2 pound pork, diced
- 1 onion, chopped & 2 fresh tomatoes, diced
- 1/3 cup chopped cilantro

Instructions

Place pinto beans in a slow cooker. Cover with water. Mix in garlic and salt. Cover, and cook 1 hour on High.

Cook the pork in a skillet over high heat until brown. Drain the fat. Place onion in the skillet. Cook until tender. Mix in jalapenos and tomatoes. Cook until heated through. Transfer to the slow cooker and stir into the beans. Continue cooking for 4 hours on Low. Mix in cilantro about half an hour before the end of the cook time.

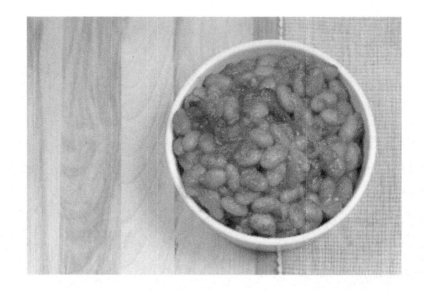

Chicken Cacciatore
Serves 8

Ingredients - Allergies: SF, GF, DF, EF, NF

- 4 pounds of chicken thighs, with skin on
- 2 Tbsp. extra virgin olive oil or avocado oil
- Salt
- 1 sliced onion
- 1/3 cup red wine
- 1 sliced red or green bell pepper
- 8 ounces sliced cremini mushrooms
- 2 sliced garlic cloves
- 3 cups peeled and chopped tomatoes
- 1 tsp. dry oregano
- 1 tsp. dry thyme
- 1 sprig fresh rosemary
- 1 tbsp. fresh parsley

Instructions

Pat the chicken on all sides with salt. Heat the olive oil in a skillet on medium. Brown few chicken pieces skin side down in the pan (don't overcrowd) for 5 minutes, then turn. Set aside. Make sure you have 2 tbsp. of the rendered fat left.

Add the onions, mushrooms and bell peppers to the pan. Increase the heat to medium high. Cook until the onions are tender, stirring, about 10 minutes. Add the garlic and cook a minute more.

Add the wine. Scrape up any browned bits and simmer until the wine is reduced by half. Add the tomatoes, pepper, oregano, thyme and a tsp. of salt. Simmer uncovered for maybe 5 more minutes. Put the chicken pieces on top of the tomatoes, skin side up. Lower the heat. Cover the skillet with the lid slightly ajar.

Cook the chicken on a low simmer. Turning and baste from time to time. Add rosemary and cook until the meat is tender, about 30 to 40 minutes. Garnish with parsley.

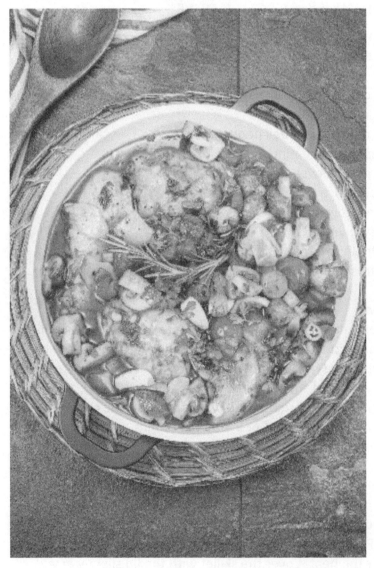

Beef Stew with Peas and Carrots

Serves 8

Ingredients - Allergies: SF, GF, DF, EF, NF

- 1-1/2 cups chopped carrots
- 1 cup chopped onions
- 2 tbsp. coconut oil
- 1-1/2 cups green peas
- 4 cups beef stock
- 1/2 tsp. salt
- 1/2 tsp. minced garlic
- 4 pounds boneless chuck roast

Instructions

Cook the onions in coconut oil on medium until they are tender (few minutes). Add all other ingredients and stir. Cover and cook on low heat for 2 hours. Mix almond flour with some cold water, add to the stew and cook for another minute.

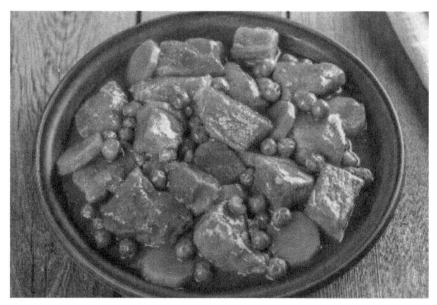

Green Chicken Stew

Serves 6-8

Ingredients - Allergies: SF, GF, DF, EF, NF

- 1-1/2 cups broccoli florets
- 1 cup chopped celery stalks
- 1 cup sliced leeks
- 2 tbsp. coconut oil
- 1-1/2 cups green peas
- 2 cups chicken stock
- 1/2 tsp. salt
- 1/2 tsp. minced garlic
- 4 pounds boneless skinless chicken pieces

Instructions

Cook the leeks in coconut oil on medium until they are tender (few minutes). Add all other ingredients and stir. Cover and cook on low heat for 1 hour. Mix almond flour with some cold water, add to the stew and cook for another minute.

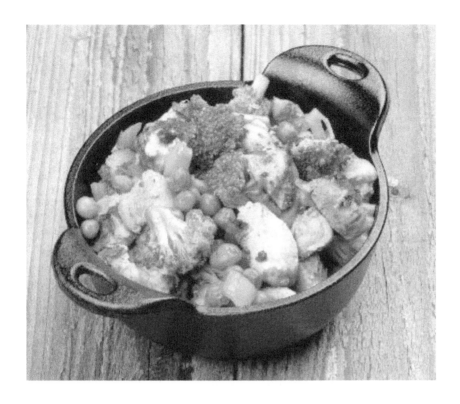

Irish Stew

Serves 8

Ingredients - Allergies: SF, GF, DF, EF, NF

- 2 chopped onions
- 2 Tbsp. coconut oil
- 1 sprig dried thyme
- 2 1/2 pounds chopped meat from lamb neck
- 6 chopped carrots
- 2 tbsp. brown rice
- 5 cups chicken stock
- Salt
- 1 bouquet garni (thyme, parsley and bay leaf)
- 2 chopped sweet potatoes
- 1 bunch chopped parsley
- 1 bunch chives

Instructions

Cook the onions in coconut oil on medium until they are tender. Add the dried thyme and lamb and stir. Add brown rice, carrots and chicken stock. Add salt, pepper and bouquet garni. Cover and cook on low heat for 2 hours. Place sweet potatoes on top of the stew and cook for 30 minutes until the meat is falling apart.

Garnish with parsley and chives.

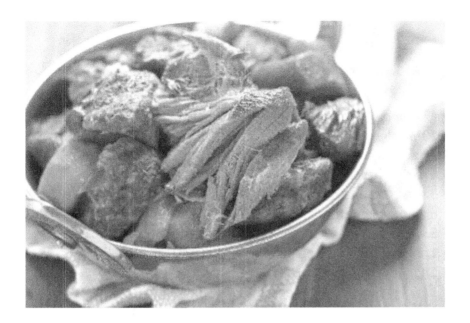

Greek Beef Stew (Stifado)

Serves 8

Ingredients - Allergies: SF, GF, DF, EF, NF

- 4 large pieces of veal or beef osso bucco
- 20 whole shallots, peeled
- 3 bay leaves
- 8 garlic cloves
- 3 sprigs rosemary
- 6 whole pimento
- 5 whole cloves
- 1/2 tsp ground nutmeg
- 1/2 cup olive oil or avocado oil
- 1/3 cup apple cider vinegar
- 1 tbsp. salt
- 2 cups tomato paste

Instructions

Mix vinegar and tomato paste and set aside. Place the meat, shallots, garlic and all spices in the pot.

Add the tomato paste, oil and vinegar. Cover the pot, bring to low boil and simmer on low for 2 hours. Do not open and stir, just shake the pot occasionally.

Serve with brown rice or maybe quinoa.

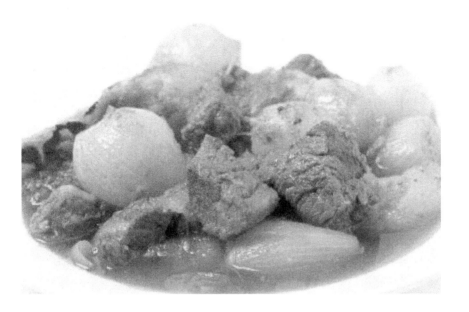

Meat Stew with Red Beans
Serves 8

Ingredients - Allergies: SF, GF, DF, EF, NF

- 3 tbsp. olive oil or avocado oil
- 1/2 chopped onion
- 1 lb lean cubed stewing beef
- 2 tsp. ground cumin
- 2 tsp. ground turmeric (optional)
- 1/2 tsp. ground cinnamon (optional)
- 2 1/2 cups water
- 5 tbsp. chopped fresh parsley
- 3 tbsp. snipped chives
- 2 cups cooked kidney beans
- 1 lemon, juice of
- 1 tbsp. almond flour

Instructions

Sauté the onion in a pan with two tablespoons of the ive oil until tender.

Add beef and cook until meat is browned on all sides. Stir in turmeric, cinnamon (both optional) and cumin and cook for one minute. Add water and bring to a boil.

Cover and simmer over low heat for 45 minutes. Stir occasionally. Sauté parsley and chives with the remaining 1 tbsp. of olive oil for about 2 minutes and add this mixture to the beef. Add kidney beans and lemon juice and season with salt and pepper.

Stir in one tbsp. of almond flour mixed with a bit of water to thicken the stew. Simmer uncovered for half an hour until meat gets tender. Serve with brown rice.

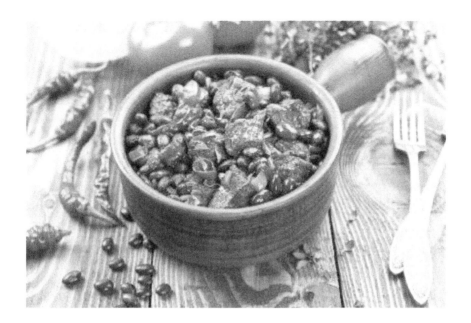

Pork Tenderloin with peppers and onions

Serves 3-4

Ingredients - Allergies: SF, GF, DF, EF, NF

- 1 tbsp. coconut oil
- 1 pound pork loin
- 1 tbsp. caraway seeds
- 1/2 tsp sea salt
- 1/4 tsp ground black pepper
- 1 red onion, thinly sliced
- 2 red bell peppers, sliced
- 2 cloves of garlic, minced
- 1/4-1/3 cup chicken broth

Instructions

Wash and chop vegetables. Slice pork loin, and season with black pepper, caraway seeds and sea salt. Heat a pan over medium heat. Add coconut oil when hot. Add pork loin and brown slightly. Add onions and mushrooms, and continue to sauté until onions are translucent. Add peppers, garlic and chicken broth. Simmer until vegetables are tender and pork is fully cooked.

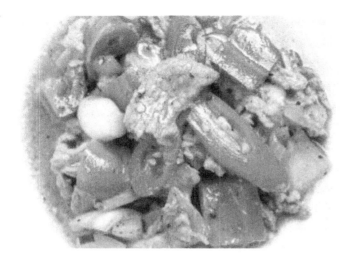

Beef Bourguinon

Serves 8-10

Ingredients - Allergies: SF, GF, DF, EF

- 4 pounds cubed lean beef
- 1 cup red wine (optional)
- 1/3 cup <u>coconut</u> oil
- 1 tsp. thyme
- 1 tsp. black pepper
- 2 cloves garlic, crushed
- 1 onion, diced
- 1 pound mushrooms, sliced
- 1 Tbsp. <u>almond</u> flour (optional)

Instructions

Marinate beef in wine, oil, thyme and pepper for few hours at room temperature or 6-8 hours in the fridge. Add beef with marinade and all other ingredients to a crock pot. Cook on low for 7-9 hrs.

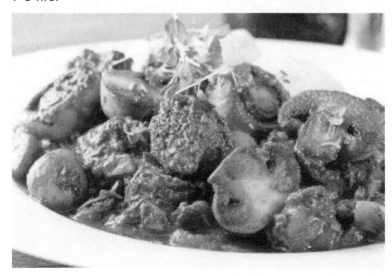

Italian Chicken

Serves 6-8

Ingredients - Allergies: SF, GF, DF, EF

- 1 skinless chicken, cut into pieces
- 1 Tbsp. almond flour (optional)
- 1 1/2 tsp. salt
- 1/8 tsp. pepper
- 1/2 cup chicken broth
- 1 cup sliced mushrooms
- 1/2 tsp. paprika
- 1 zucchini, sliced into medium pieces
- ground black pepper
- parsley to garnish

Instructions

Season chicken with 1 tsp. salt. Combine flour, pepper, remaining salt, and paprika. Coat chicken pieces with this mixture. Place zucchini first in a crockpot. Pour broth over zucchini. Arrange chicken on top. Cover and cook on low for 6 to 8 hours or until tender. Turn control to high, add mushrooms, cover, and cook on high for additional 10-15 minutes. Garnish with parsley and ground black pepper.

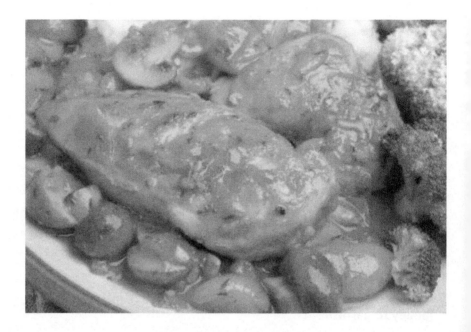

Ropa Vieja

Ingredients - Allergies: SF, GF, DF, EF, NF

6 servings

- 1 tbsp. coconut oil
- 2 pounds beef flank steak
- 1 cup beef broth
- 1 cup tomato sauce
- 1 small onion, sliced
- 1 green bell pepper sliced into strips
- 2 cloves garlic, chopped
- 1/2 cup tomato paste
- 1 tsp. ground cumin
- 1 tsp. chopped cilantro
- 1 tbsp. olive oil & 1 tbsp. lemon juice

Instructions

Add all ingredients to a crock pot. Cover, and cook on high for 4 hours, or on Low for up to 8 hours.

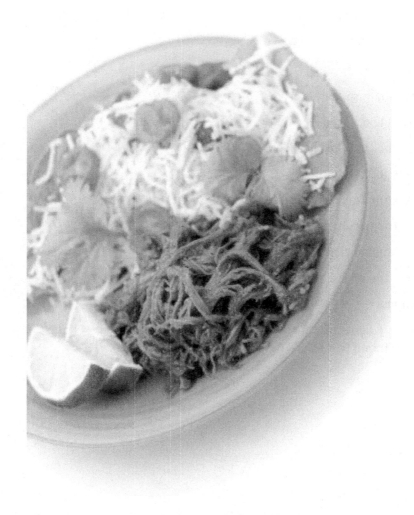

Lemon Roast Chicken

Serves 6-8

Ingredients - Allergies: SF, GF, DF, EF, NF

- 1 whole skinless chicken
- 1 dash Salt
- 1 dash Pepper
- 1 tsp. Oregano
- 2 cloves minced garlic
- 2 tbsp. coconut oil
- 1/4 cup Water
- 3 tbsp. Lemon juice
- Rosemary

Instructions

Add ingredients to a crock pot and cover. Cook on low 7 hours. Add lemon juice when cooking is done.

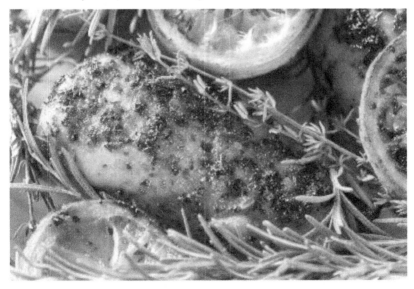

Fall Lamb and Vegetable Stew

Serves 6-8

Ingredients - Allergies: SF, GF, DF, EF, NF

- 2 pounds Lamb stew meat
- 1 chopped Tomato
- 1 cup green beans
- 1 cup carrots, sliced
- 1/2 cup green peas
- 1 cup Onions, chopped
- 2 teaspoons Salt
- 1 each Garlic cloves, crushed
- 1/2 tsp. Thyme leaves
- 1 each Bay leaves
- 2 cups chicken broth

Instructions

Cut green beans. Place vegetables and lamb in crockpot. Mix salt, garlic, thyme, and bay leaf into broth and pour over lamb and vegetables. Cover and cook on low for 7 hours.

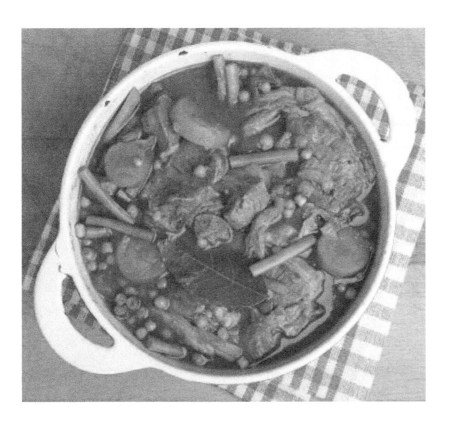

Slow cooker pork loin

Serves 4-6

Ingredients - Allergies: SF, GF, DF, EF, NF

- 1-1/2 lb pork loin

- 1 cup tomato sauce

- 2 zucchinis, sliced

- 1 head cauliflower, separated into medium florets

- 1-2 Tbs dried basil

- 1/4 tsp ground black pepper

- 1/2 tsp sea salt (optional)

Instructions

Add all of the ingredients to a crock pot.

Cook on high for 3-4 hours or low 7-8 hours.

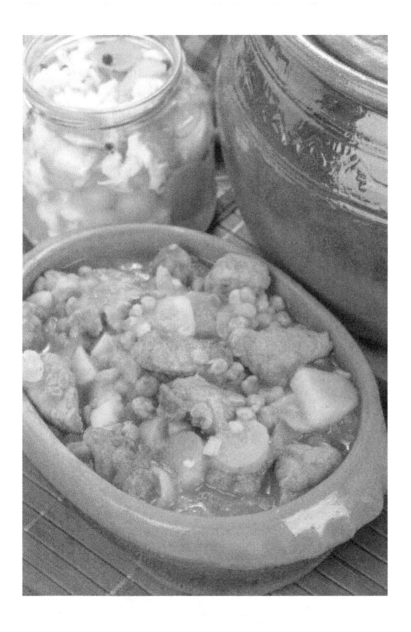

Pork, Zucchini, Pork, Tomato & Corn Stew

Serves 8

Ingredients - Allergies: SF, GF, DF, EF, NF

- 1/2 cups cooked corn (optional)
- 1 cup chopped onions
- 1-1/2 cups sliced zucchini
- 1 cup chopped tomato
- 2 tbsp. coconut oil
- 2 tbsp. chopped garlic
- 2 tsp. salt and 1 tsp. ground pepper
- 4 pounds cubed pork

Instructions

Put ingredients in the slow cooker. Cover, and cook on low for 7 to 9 hours.

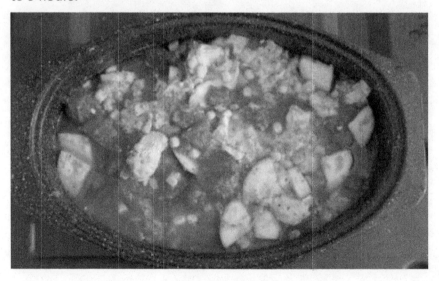

Red Peppers Pork Curry

Serves 8

Ingredients - Allergies: SF, GF, DF, EF, NF

- 3 cups sliced red peppers
- 1 cup chopped onions
- 2 tbsp. coconut oil
- 1 cup curry paste*
- 4 pounds chopped pork meat

Instructions

Put ingredients in the slow cooker. Cover, and cook on low for 7 to 9 hours.

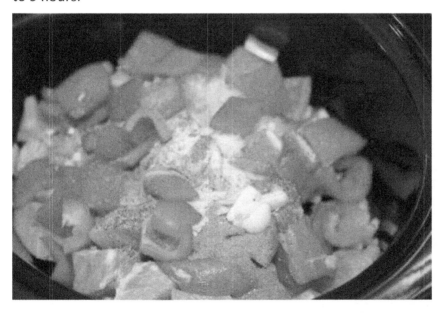

Beef Ratatouille

Serves 8

Ingredients - Allergies: SF, GF, DF, EF, NF

- 1-1/2 cups sliced zucchini
- 1 cup chopped onions
- 1-1/2 cups sliced eggplant
- 1-1/2 cups sliced red peppers (or tomato)
- 2 tbsp. coconut oil
- 2 tbsp. chopped garlic
- 2 tsp. salt and 1 tsp. ground pepper
- 4 pounds cubed beef

Instructions

Put ingredients in the slow cooker. Cover, and cook on low for 7 to 9 hours.

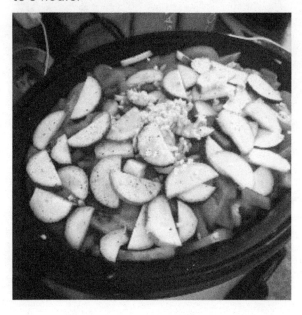

Brown Rice Dishes
Serves 4-6

Paella

Ingredients - Allergies: SF, GF, DF, EF, NF

- 1 onion, finely chopped
- 5 tbsp. coconut oil
- 2 chopped garlic clove
- 2 chopped tomatoes
- Salt
- 1 tsp. sweet paprika
- A pinch of saffron
- 4 cleaned small squid, sliced
- 2 cups medium-grain brown rice
- 3 cups fish or chicken broth, plus more if needed
- 1 cup dry white wine
- 12 jumbo shrimps
- 16 mussels, scrubbed and debearded

Instructions

Put the oil in a 16-inch paella pan and fry the onion until soft. Stir in the garlic and tomatoes. Add salt to taste, paprika, and saffron, stir well, and cook until the tomatoes get soft. Add the squid and the rice and stir well.

Bring the wine and broth to a boil in a saucepan. Pour over the rice, bring to a boil, and add salt. Spread the rice in the pan. Cook the rice over low heat for 20 minutes. Put the shrimp on top after 10 minutes. Once they become pin, turn them. When the rice is done, turn off the heat and cover the pan.

Steam the mussels and put them on top of the paella.

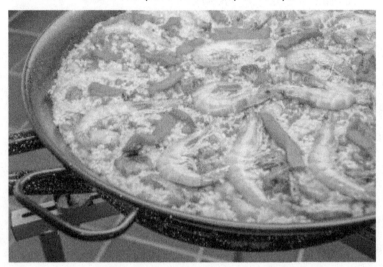

Asparagus Mint Lemon Risotto

Serves 6-8

Ingredients - Allergies: SF, GF, DF, EF, NF

For the risotto base

- 1 liter vegetable or chicken broth
- 2 tbsp. olive oil or cumin oil
- 1 large onion, peeled and finely chopped
- 4-5 sticks celery, trimmed and finely chopped
- 600 g brown rice
- 250 ml dry white wine

For the risotto

- 2 bunches asparagus, woody ends removed and discarded
- 700 ml vegetable or chicken broth
- 50 g coconut oil
- 1 bunch fresh mint, leaves picked and finely chopped
- zest and juice of 2 lemons
- sea salt
- extra virgin olive oil or avocado oil

Instructions

Chop asparagus discs, keeping the tips whole. Bring the broth to a simmer in a saucepan. Put the olive oil in a separate pan, add the celery and the onion and cook until soft. Add the rice and wine and turn up the heat and keep stirring.

Add the broth to the rice a ladle at a time, stir well and wait until it has been absorbed. When it's all absorbed, put to one side. Put a saucepan on high heat and pour in half the broth, followed by all risotto base and the asparagus. Simmer until almost all the broth has been absorbed. Add the rest of the broth in batches until the rice and asparagus are cooked. Turn off the heat, add olive oil, mint, lemon zest and all the juice. Check the seasoning and add salt and pepper if needed.

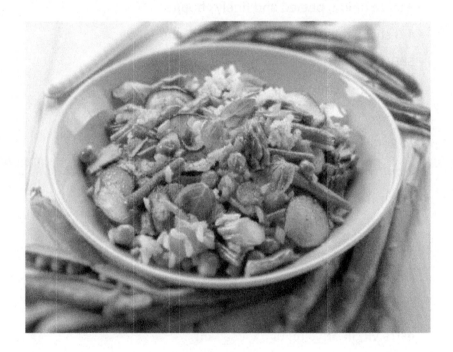

Stir Fries

Pork and Bok Choy / Celery Stir Fry

Serves 1 - Allergies: SF, GF, DF, EF, NF

5 oz. Lean Pork Tenderloin and Bok Choy / Celery stir fry. Use as much veggies as you want or replace Bok Choy with Kale. Season with fish sauce.

Nutrition Facts

Serving Size 574 g

Amount Per Serving

Calories 316   Calories from Fat 39

% Daily Value*

Total Fat 4.3g	**7%**
Saturated Fat 1.1g	**6%**
Trans Fat 0.0g	
Cholesterol 82mg	**27%**
Sodium 1156mg	**48%**
Potassium 1314mg	**38%**
Total Carbohydrates 34.6g	**12%**
Dietary Fiber 8.8g	**35%**
Sugars 8.8g	
Protein 34.5g	

Vitamin A 33%	Vitamin C 81%
Calcium 9%	Iron 30%

Nutrition Grade A

* Based on a 2000 calorie diet

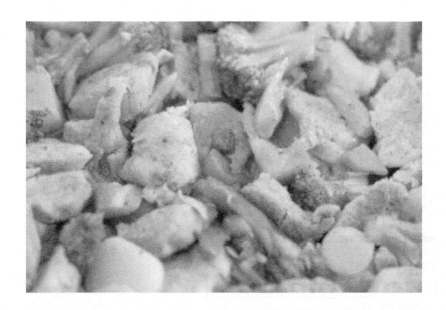

Lemon Chicken Stir Fry

Serves 3-4

Ingredients - Allergies: SF, GF, DF, EF, NF

- 1 lemon

- 1/2 cup chicken broth

- 3 tbsp. fish sauce

- 2 teaspoons arrowroot flour

- 1 tbsp. coconut oil

- 1 pound boneless, skinless chicken breasts, trimmed and cut into 1-inch pieces

- 10 ounces mushrooms, halved or quartered

- 2 cups snow peas, stems and strings removed

- 1 bunch scallions, cut into 1-inch pieces, white and green parts divided

- 1 tbsp. chopped garlic

Instructions

Grate 1 tsp. lemon zest. Juice the lemon and mix 3 tbsp. of the juice with broth, fish sauce and arrowroot flour in a small bowl.

Heat oil in a skillet over high heat. Add chicken and cook, stirring occasionally, until just cooked through. Transfer to a plate. Add mushrooms to the pan and cook until the mushrooms are tender. Add snow peas, garlic, scallion whites and the lemon zest. Cook, stirring, around 30 seconds. Add the broth to the pan and cook, stirring, 2 to 3 minutes. Add scallion greens and the chicken and any accumulated juices and stir.

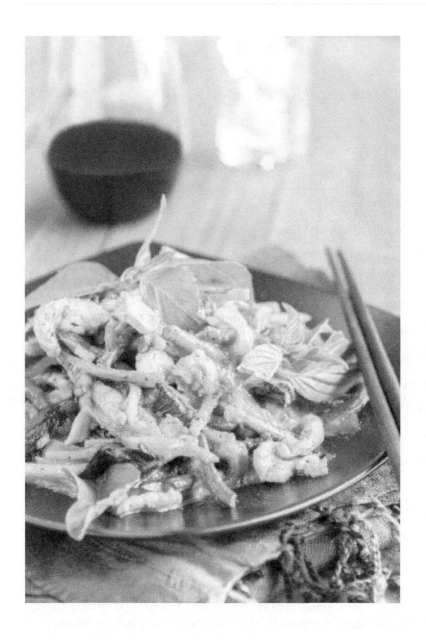

Beef and Broccoli Stir Fry
Serves 1 - Allergies: SF, GF, DF, EF, NF

• 5oz. of lean Beef and 1 cup broccoli stir fry. Use as much broccoli as you want or replace Broccoli with Kale.

Nutrition Facts

Serving Size 251 g

Amount Per Serving

Calories 342   Calories from Fat 124

	% Daily Value*
Total Fat 13.8g	**21%**
Saturated Fat 4.0g	**20%**
Trans Fat 0.0g	
Cholesterol 127mg	**42%**
Sodium 1024mg	**43%**
Potassium 884mg	**25%**
Total Carbohydrates 7.0g	**2%**
Dietary Fiber 2.4g	**10%**
Sugars 1.7g	
Protein 46.5g	

Vitamin A 11%	•	Vitamin C 131%
Calcium 5%	•	Iron 154%

Nutrition Grade A-
* Based on a 2000 calorie diet

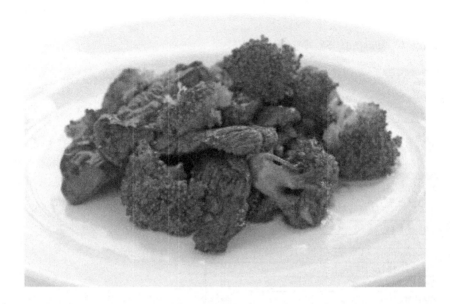

Thai Basil Chicken

Serves 1

Ingredients - Allergies: SF, GF, DF, NF

For the egg

- 1 egg
- 2 tbsp. of coconut oil for frying

Basil chicken

- 1 chicken breast (or any other cut of boneless chicken, about 200 grams)
- 5 cloves of garlic
- 4 Thai chilies
- 1 tbsp. coconut oil for frying
- Fish sauce
- 1 handful of Thai holy basil leaves

Instructions

First, fry the egg.

Basil chicken

Cut the chicken into small pieces. Peel the garlic and chilies, and chop them fine. Add basil leaves.

Add about 1 tbsp. of oil to the pan.

When the oil is hot, add the chilies and garlic. Stir fry for half a minute.

Toss in your chicken and keep stir frying. Add fish sauce.

Add basil into the pan, fold it into the chicken, and turn off the heat.

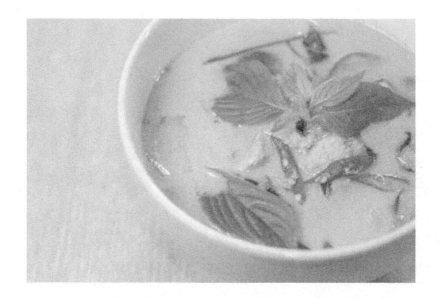

Shrimp with Snow Peas

Serves 4.

Ingredients - Allergies: SF, GF, DF, EF, NF

Marinade

- 2 teaspoons arrowroot flour
- 1 Tbsp wine
- 1/2 tsp. salt

Stir Fry

- 1 pound shrimp, peeled and deveined
- 2 Tbsp coconut oil
- 1 Tbsp minced ginger
- 3 garlic cloves, sliced thinly
- 1/2 pound snow peas, strings removed
- 2 teaspoons fish sauce
- 1/4 cup chicken broth
- 4 green onions, white and light green parts, sliced diagonally
- 2 teaspoons dark roasted sesame oil

Instructions

Mix all the ingredients for the marinade in a bowl and then add the shrimp. Mix to coat. Let it marinade 15 minutes while you prepare the peas, ginger, and garlic.

Add the coconut oil in the wok and let it get hot. Add the garlic and ginger and combine. Stir-fry for about 30 seconds.

Add the marinade to the wok, add the snow peas, fish sauce and chicken broth. Stir-fry until the shrimp turns pink. Add the green onions and stir-fry for one more minute. Turn off the heat and add the sesame oil. Toss once more and serve with steamed brown rice or soba gluten free noodles.

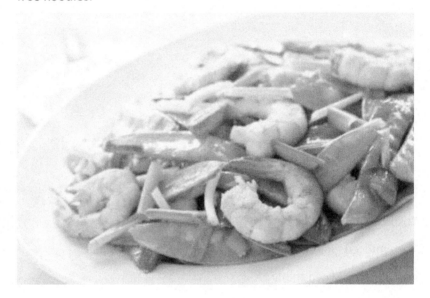

Pork and Green Beans Stir Fry

Serves 1 - Allergies: SF, GF, DF, EF, NF

- 6oz. of lean Pork

- 1 cup of Green Beans, snapped in half. Use as much veggies as you want or replace Green beans with Kale.

- 1 garlic clove, chopped

- 1/2 inch of peeled and chopped ginger

- Season with fish sauce.

Nutrition Facts

Serving Size 285 g

Amount Per Serving

Calories 317	Calories from Fat 97
	% Daily Value*
Total Fat 10.8g	17%
Saturated Fat 2.7g	14%
Trans Fat 0.1g	
Cholesterol 124mg	41%
Sodium 104mg	4%
Potassium 946mg	27%
Total Carbohydrates 7.8g	3%
Dietary Fiber 3.7g	15%
Sugars 1.5g	
Protein 46.5g	

Vitamin A 15%	•	Vitamin C 30%
Calcium 5%	•	Iron 17%

Nutrition Grade A

* Based on a 2000 calorie diet

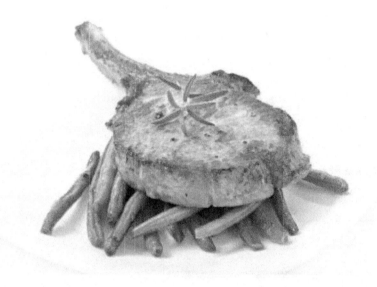

Cashew chicken

Serves 4

Ingredients - Allergies: SF, GF, DF, EF, NF

- 1 bunch scallions
- 1 pound skinless boneless chicken thighs
- 1/2 tsp. salt
- 3 tbsp. coconut oil
- 1 red bell pepper and 1 stalk of celery, chopped
- 4 garlic cloves, finely chopped
- 1 1/2 tbsp. finely chopped peeled fresh ginger
- 1/4 tsp. dried hot red-pepper flakes
- 3/4 cup chicken broth
- 1 1/2 tbsp. fish sauce
- 1 1/2 teaspoons arrowroot flour
- 1/2 cup salted roasted whole cashews

Instructions

Chop scallions and separate green and white parts. Pat chicken dry and cut into 3/4-inch pieces and season with salt and pepper. Heat a wok or a skillet over high heat. Add oil and then stir-fry chicken until cooked through, 3 to 4 minutes. Transfer to a plate. Add garlic, bell pepper, celery, ginger, red-pepper flakes, and scallion whites to wok and stir-fry until peppers are just tender, 4 to 5 minutes.

Mix together broth, fish sauce and arrowroot flour, then stir into vegetables in wok. Reduce heat and simmer, stirring occasionally, until thickened. Stir in cashews, scallion greens, and chicken along with any juices.

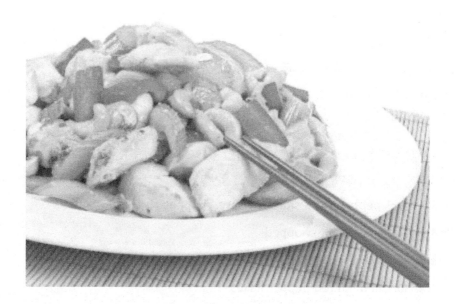

Meats

Baked Chicken Breast with Fresh Basil

Serves 10

Ingredients - Allergies: SF, GF, EF, NF

- 10 boneless skinless chicken breast
- 3/4 cup low-fat yogurt
- 1/2 cup chopped basil
- 2 tsp. arrowroot flour
- 1 cup oatmeal coarsely ground

Instructions

Arrange chicken in a baking dish. Combine basil, yogurt and arrowroot flour; mix well and spread over chicken.

Mix oatmeal with salt and pepper to taste and sprinkle over chicken.

Bake chicken in 375 degrees in the oven for half an hour. Makes 10 servings.

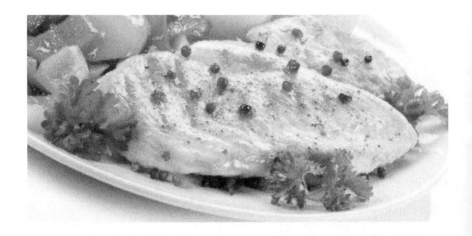

Roast Chicken with Rosemary
Serves 6-8

- 1 (3 pound) whole chicken, rinsed, skinned
- salt and pepper to taste
- 1 onion, quartered
- 1/4 cup chopped rosemary

Instructions - Allergies: SF, GF, DF, EF, NF

Heat the oven to 350F. Sprinkle salt and pepper on meat. Stuff with the onion and rosemary. Place in a baking dish and bake in the preheated oven until chicken is cooked through. Depending on the size of the bird, cooking time will vary.

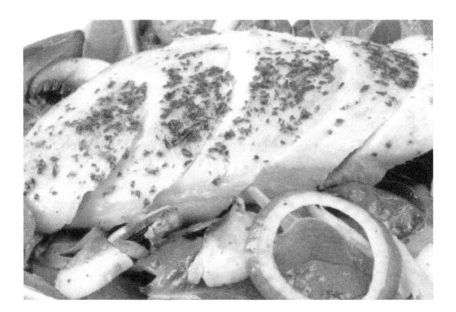

Carne Asada

Serves 4- Allergies: SF, GF, DF, EF, NF

Ingredients:
- 2 pounds of flank steak
- 2 cloves garlic, chopped
- 1/2 cup of chopped cilantro
- 1 tsp. salt
- 2 Tbsp. Olive oil
- 1 lime, squeezed juice
- 1 orange, squeezed juice

Mix together the garlic, jalapeno, cilantro, salt, and pepper to make a paste. Put the paste in a container. Add the oil, lime juice and orange juice. Shake it up to combine. Use as a marinade for beef or as a table condiment.

Instructions

Put the flank steak in a baking dish and pour the marinade over it. Refrigerate up to 8 hours.
Take the steak out of the marinade and season it on both sides with salt and pepper. Grill (or broil) the steak for 7 to 10 minutes per side, turning once, until medium-rare. Put the steak on a cutting board and allow the juices to settle (5 minutes). Thinly

slice the steak across the grain.

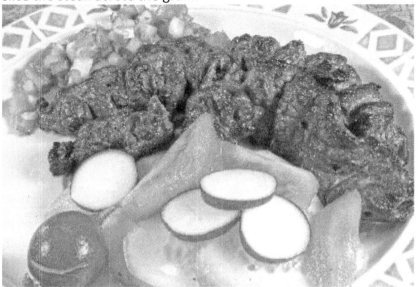

Meatballs

Baked Beef Meatballs

This amount is for 4 servings. Adjust for 2 if you want, eat one serving, freeze one or prepare it as is for 4 servings and then freeze 3/4 for some tasty casserole recipes like "Beef Meatballs Casserole with Green Beans" or with "Beef Meatballs Casserole with Broccoli".

Allergies: SF, GF, NF

- 1 pound lean ground beef
- 2 tbsp. minced onion
- 1/2 tsp. minced garlic
- 1 tsp. parmesan cheese
- 2 eggs
- 1/2 tsp. salt
- 1/4 tsp. pepper

Mix all of the ingredients in a large bowl using your fingers. Mix until the meat no long feels slimy from the eggs. Shape in small egg size meatballs. Place on a baking sheet. Bake at 375F for 20-25 minutes until the meatballs are cooked through. Serve with large Fiber Loaded salad

Nutrition Facts

Serving Size 149 g

Amount Per Serving

Calories 268	Calories from Fat 97

% Daily Value*

Total Fat 10.8g	**17%**
Saturated Fat 4.3g	**22%**
Trans Fat 0.0g	
Cholesterol 188mg	**63%**
Sodium 461mg	**19%**
Potassium 497mg	**14%**
Total Carbohydrates 1.1g	**0%**
Protein 39.5g	

Vitamin A 3%	•	Vitamin C 1%
Calcium 8%	•	Iron 121%

Nutrition Grade B

* Based on a 2000 calorie diet

with Italian Dressing.

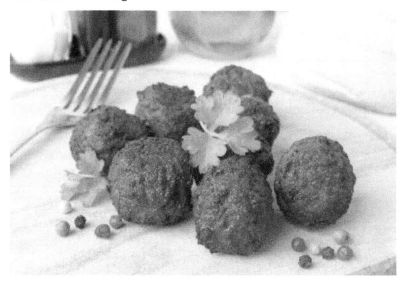

Middle Eastern Meatballs

Makes about 20 meatballs - Allergies: SF, GF, DF, EF, NF

Ingredients

- Ground lamb or beef, or a mixture of the two -- 2 pounds
- Onion, minced -- 1
- Fresh parsley or mint, finely chopped -- 1/2 bunch
- Ground cumin -- 1 tbsp.
- Cinnamon -- 2 teaspoons
- Allspice (optional) -- 1 tsp.
- Salt and pepper -- to season
- <u>coconut</u> oil -- 1/4 cup

Instructions

Place the ground beef or lamb, onion, herbs, spices, salt and pepper in a bowl and knead well. Chill for 1-2 hours and let the flavors mingle. Form the meat into patties or balls the size of a small egg.

Bake in the oven on 350F. Serve with brown rice with tzatziki sauce.

Variations

Experiment with different seasonings--coriander, cayenne, sesame seeds.

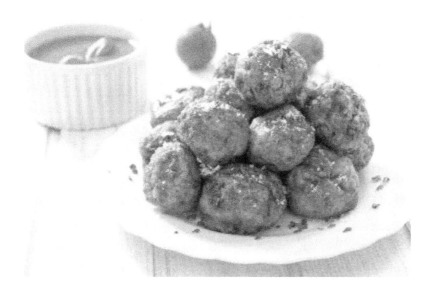

Casseroles

Some recipes are for 1 person, adjust for 2 or more

Broccoli Chicken Casserole

Serves 1

Ingredients - Allergies: SF, GF, NF

• 1 cup broccoli florets

• 6 oz. skinless, boneless chicken (or turkey) pieces (breast or dark meat)

• 1 tsp of <u>flax</u> seeds meal

• Salt, pepper

• 1 egg - beaten

• Half a cup of Yogurt Dressing (or coconut milk, if you don't like the sourish tang)

• 1/4 cup of chicken broth

• 2 tbsp of grated low-fat cheddar cheese

Heat the oven to 400°. Cook broccoli around 5 minutes. Take broccoli out and add chicken (or turkey) and simmer for 15 minutes. Cut chicken (or turkey) into cubes and add it to the broccoli.

Combine broth, flax, salt and pepper in a pan and mix. Bring to a boil over high heat and cook 1 minute, stirring constantly. Remove from heat. Add yogurt dressing, beaten egg and then half of the cheese, stirring until well combined. Add sauce to broccoli mixture; and stir gently until combined.

Put mixture in a small casserole dish oiled with some coconut oil. Put remaining cheese on top, sprinkle. Bake at 400° for 50 minutes or until mixture bubbles at the edges and cheese begins to brown. Remove from oven and let cool for 5 minutes.

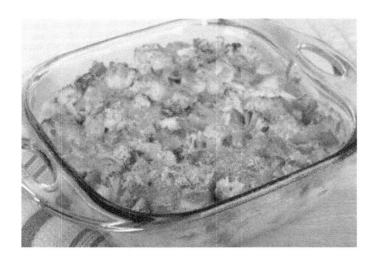

Beef Meatballs Broccoli Casserole

Serves 1

Ingredients - Allergies: SF, GF

- 1 cup broccoli florets
- 4 oz. beef meatballs (see separate recipe)
- 1 tsp of almond flour
- Salt, pepper
- 1 egg - beaten
- Half a cup of Yogurt Dressing
- 1/4 cup of chicken broth
- 2 tbsp of grated low-fat cheddar cheese

Instructions

Heat oven to 400F. Cook broccoli around 5 minutes. Prepare beef meatballs as in the recipe above. Combine broth, flour, salt and pepper in a saucepan, stirring with a whisk until smooth. Bring to a boil over medium-high heat; cook 1 minute, stirring constantly. Remove from heat. Add yogurt dressing, beaten egg and then half of the cheese, stirring until well combined. Add sauce to broccoli mixture; and stir gently until combined.

Put mixture in a small casserole dish oiled with some coconut oil. Sprinkle with remaining cheese. Bake at 400° for 50 minutes or until mixture bubbles at the edges and cheese begins to brown. Remove from oven and let cool for 5 minutes. Serve with large Fiber Loaded Salad with Italian Dressing.

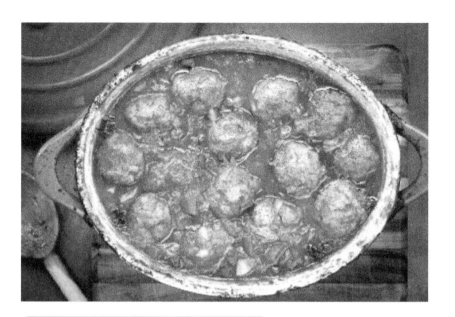

Nutrition Facts

Serving Size 352 g

Amount Per Serving

Calories 409   Calories from Fat 147

	% Daily Value*
Total Fat 16.3g	**25%**
Saturated Fat 6.5g	**32%**
Trans Fat 0.0g	
Cholesterol 277mg	**92%**
Sodium 745mg	**31%**
Potassium 958mg	**27%**
Total Carbohydrates 11.2g	**4%**
Dietary Fiber 2.2g	**9%**
Sugars 6.2g	
Protein 52.0g	

Vitamin A 29%	•	Vitamin C 104%
Calcium 30%	•	Iron 128%

Nutrition Grade A-

* Based on a 2000 calorie diet

Beef Meatballs Cauliflower Casserole

Serves 1

Ingredients - Allergies: SF, GF

- 1 cup cauliflower florets
- 4 oz. beef meatballs (see separate recipe)
- 1 tsp of <u>almond</u> flour
- Salt, pepper
- 1 egg - beaten
- Half a cup of Yogurt Dressing
- 1/4 cup of chicken broth
- 2 tbsp of grated low-fat cheddar cheese

Instructions

Heat oven to 400°.

Cook cauliflower around 5 minutes. Prepare beef meatballs as in the recipe above. Combine soup, flour, salt and pepper in a saucepan, stirring with a whisk until smooth. Bring to a boil over medium-high heat; cook 1 minute, stirring constantly. Remove from heat. Add yogurt dressing, beaten egg and then half of the cheese, stirring until well combined. Add sauce to cauliflower mixture; and stir gently until combined.

Put mixture in a small casserole dish oiled with some coconut oil. Sprinkle with remaining cheese. Bake at 400° for 50 minutes or until mixture bubbles at the edges and cheese begins to brown. Remove from oven and let cool for 5 minutes. Serve with large Fiber Loaded Salad with Italian Dressing.

Nutrition Facts

Serving Size 361 g

Amount Per Serving

Calories 405   Calories from Fat 145

	% Daily Value*
Total Fat 16.1g	**25%**
Saturated Fat 6.5g	**32%**
Trans Fat 0.0g	
Cholesterol 277mg	**92%**
Sodium 745mg	**31%**
Potassium 976mg	**28%**
Total Carbohydrates 10.8g	**4%**
Dietary Fiber 2.3g	**9%**
Sugars 6.9g	
Protein 51.6g	

Vitamin A 21%	•	Vitamin C 64%
Calcium 28%	•	Iron 127%

Nutrition Grade A-

* Based on a 2000 calorie diet

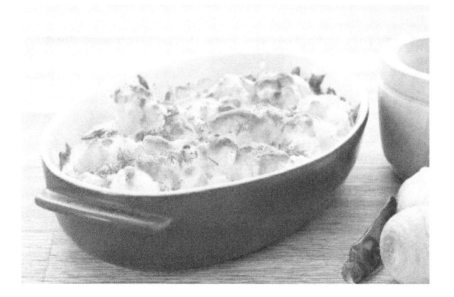

Cabbage Roll Casserole

Serves 8

Ingredients - Allergies: SF, GF, DF, EF, NF

2 pounds ground beef
1 cup chopped onion
1 liter tomato sauce
3 1/2 pounds cabbage or sauerkraut leaves
1 cup uncooked brown rice
1 tsp. salt
2 cups beef broth

Instructions

Heat oven to 350F.
Brown beef in coconut oil in a skillet over medium high heat until through. In a large mixing bowl combine the onion, rice and salt. Add meat and mix all together. Roll mixture into cabbage leaves and arrange them in a casserole dish. Pour broth and tomato sauce over rolls and bake in the preheated oven, covered, for 1 hour.

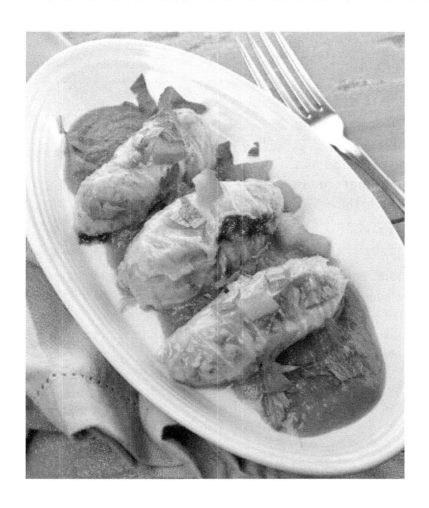

Pork Chop Casserole

Serves 6

Ingredients - Allergies: SF, GF, DF, EF, NF

- 3 cups vegetable broth
- 1 cup brown rice
- 5 ounce mushrooms
- salt and pepper to taste
- 6 (3/4 inch) thick pork chops

Instructions

Heat oven to 350F. Pour broth into a baking dish. Add rice and mushrooms and mix. Salt and pepper to taste. Add pork chops in a single layer on that mixture and push them down into mixture and make sure they are covered with it.
Cover baking dish with aluminum foil and bake for 1 hour.

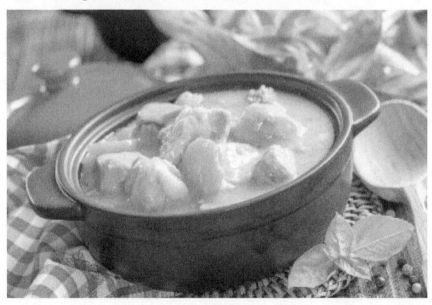

Mushrooms Casserole

Instructions – serves 4 - Allergies: SF, GF, NF

- 3 pounds sliced mushrooms (shiitake preferably)

- 1 pound sliced leeks

- Salt

- 1 tbsp. chopped parsley

- 2 beaten eggs

- 1 cup of low-fat Greek yogurt

- 1/2 cup of shredded cheddar cheese, low-fat

- 1 pound cubed skinless boneless chicken (or turkey) breasts

Instructions

Heat oven to 375 degrees F. Mix beaten eggs and low-fat yogurt in a separate dish. In a casserole, place 1 layer of mushrooms, leeks and chicken cubes and season with salt, pepper, and parsley. Cover with 1/2 of a cup of eggs/yogurt mixture. Repeat process 2 more times and cover with shredded cheese. Bake until mushrooms and chicken is tender and crust is golden brown. Serve with Large Fiber Loaded salad with Italian Dressing.

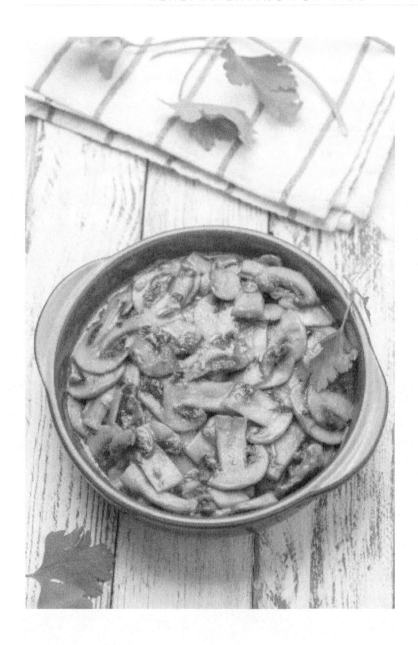

Nutrition Facts

Serving Size 647 g

Amount Per Serving

Calories 325	Calories from Fat 55
	% Daily Value*

Total Fat 6.1g	**9%**
Saturated Fat 1.7g	**9%**
Trans Fat 0.0g	
Cholesterol 143mg	**48%**
Sodium 520mg	**22%**
Potassium 1426mg	**41%**
Total Carbohydrates 30.8g	**10%**
Dietary Fiber 5.5g	**22%**
Sugars 13.5g	
Protein 44.9g	

Vitamin A 41%	Vitamin C 43%
Calcium 23%	Iron 74%

Nutrition Grade A

* Based on a 2000 calorie diet

Beef Meatballs Green Beans Casserole

Serves 1

Ingredients - Allergies: SF, GF

- 1 cup green beans florets
- 5 oz. beef meatballs (see separate recipe)
- 1 tsp of almond flour
- Salt, pepper
- 1 egg - beaten

Half a cup of Yogurt Dressing

- 1/4 cup of chicken broth
- 2 tbsp. of grated low-fat cheddar cheese

Instructions

Heat oven to 400°.

Cook green beans around 5 minutes. Prepare beef meatballs as in the recipe above. Combine soup, flour, salt and pepper in a saucepan, stirring with a whisk until smooth. Bring to a boil over medium-high heat; cook 1 minute, stirring constantly. Remove from heat. Add yogurt dressing, beaten egg and then half of the cheese, stirring until well combined. Add sauce to green beans mixture; and stir gently until combined.

Put mixture in a small casserole dish oiled with some coconut oil. Sprinkle with remaining cheese. Bake at 400° for 50 minutes or until mixture bubbles at the edges and cheese begins to brown. Remove from oven and let cool for 5 minutes. Serve with large Fiber Loaded Salad with Italian Dressing.

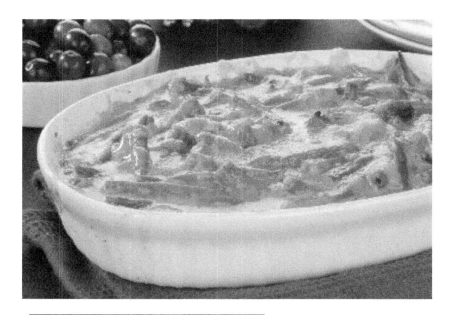

Nutrition Facts

Serving Size 368 g

Amount Per Serving

Calories 412   Calories from Fat 146

	% Daily Value*
Total Fat 16.2g	**25%**
Saturated Fat 6.5g	**32%**
Trans Fat 0.0g	
Cholesterol 277mg	**92%**
Sodium 728mg	**30%**
Potassium 921mg	**26%**
Total Carbohydrates 12.7g	**4%**
Dietary Fiber 3.3g	**13%**
Sugars 6.2g	
Protein 51.6g	

Vitamin A 32%	•	Vitamin C 28%
Calcium 30%	•	Iron 130%

Nutrition Grade A-

* Based on a 2000 calorie diet

"Breaded" "fried" food
Breaded Tilapia

Ingredients - Allergies: SF, GF, DF, NF

Recipe is for 4 servings.

- 1 cup coconut meal for breading
- 1/2 tsp. pepper
- 1/2 tsp. minced garlic
- 1/2 tsp. paprika
- 1/4 tsp. salt
- 2 large egg whites (or whole eggs), beaten
- 1 pound tilapia fillets, cut into 1/2-by-3-inch strips

Instructions

Heat oven to 400°F. Set a wire rack on a baking sheet and coat with some coconut oil.

Place coconut, pepper, garlic, paprika and salt in a blender and process until finely ground. Transfer to a shallow dish.

Place egg whites in a second dish. Dip every piece of fish in the egg and then coat all sides with the coconut breading mixture. Place on the prepared rack. Sprinkle some drops of olive oil over each piece.

Bake until the fish is cooked through. Breading should be golden brown. Serve with large Fiber loaded salad.

Nutrition Facts

Serving Size 189 g

Amount Per Serving

Calories 261	Calories from Fat 130
	% Daily Value*
Total Fat 14.4g	**22%**
Saturated Fat 1.3g	**7%**
Trans Fat 0.0g	
Cholesterol 137mg	**46%**
Sodium 227mg	**9%**
Potassium 103mg	**3%**
Total Carbohydrates 9.6g	**3%**
Dietary Fiber 8.6g	**34%**
Sugars 0.8g	
Protein 30.3g	

Vitamin A 17%	•	Vitamin C 14%
Calcium 9%	•	Iron 18%

Nutrition Grade B-

* Based on a 2000 calorie diet

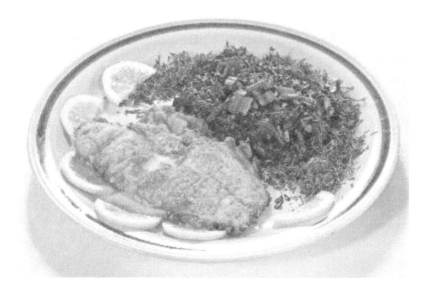

Breaded Chicken

Ingredients - Allergies: SF, GF, DF, NF

Recipe is for 4 servings.

- 1 cup flax seeds meal for breading
- 1/2 tsp. pepper
- 1/2 tsp. minced garlic
- 1/2 tsp. paprika
- 1/4 tsp. salt
- 2 large egg whites (or whole eggs), beaten
- 1 pound skinless, boneless chicken pieces

Instructions

Heat oven to 400°F. Set a wire rack on a baking sheet; coat with some coconut oil.

Place flax, pepper, garlic, paprika and salt in a food processor or blender and process until finely ground. Transfer to a shallow dish.

Place egg whites in a second dish. Dip every piece of chicken in the egg and then coat all sides with the flax breading mixture. Place on the prepared rack. Sprinkle some drops of olive oil over each piece.

Bake until the chicken is cooked through and the breading is golden brown and crisp, about 8 minutes each side. Serve with large Fiber loaded salad.

Nutrition Facts

Serving Size 189 g

Amount Per Serving

Calories 384   Calories from Fat 196

	% Daily Value*
Total Fat 21.8g	**34%**
Saturated Fat 3.2g	**16%**
Trans Fat 0.0g	
Cholesterol 183mg	**61%**
Sodium 285mg	**12%**
Potassium 378mg	**11%**
Total Carbohydrates 9.6g	**3%**
Dietary Fiber 8.6g	**34%**
Sugars 0.8g	
Protein 42.0g	

Vitamin A 18%	•	Vitamin C 14%
Calcium 8%	•	Iron 19%

Nutrition Grade B+

* Based on a 2000 calorie diet

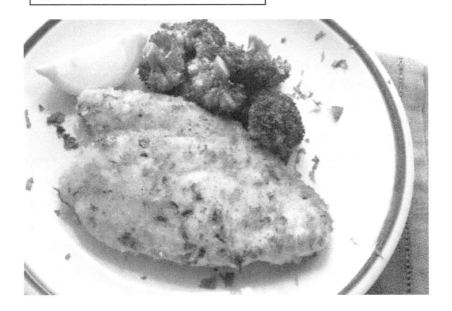

Lemon Pork with Asparagus

Serves: 3-4

Ingredients - Allergies: SF, GF, DF, EF, NF

- 1 lb. pork chops
- 1/4 cup buckwheat flour
- 1/2 tsp. salt
- 2 tbsp. coconut oil
- Pepper
- 1 cup chopped asparagus
- 2 lemons, sliced

Instructions

Place the flour and salt in a dish and gently toss each chop in the dish to coat. Melt the coconut oil in a large skillet over medium high heat. Add the chicken and sauté until golden brown on each side. Sprinkle each side with the pepper directly in the pan.

When the chops are cooked through, transfer them to a plate. Add the lemon slices and asparagus to the pan. When the asparagus and the lemons are done, add the chops back to the pan.

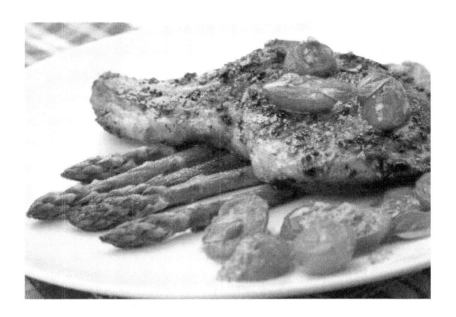

Pizza
Meat Pizza

Serves 4

Ingredients - Allergies: SF, GF, EF, NF

- 1 cup cooked and minced chicken breast
- 1 cup low-fat cheddar, shredded
- 1 tbsp. minced onion & few basil leaves
- 1 tsp garlic minced

Instructions

Preheat oven to 425 degrees Fahrenheit. Process chicken, onion and garlic together. Mixture will be a dense crumb consistency. Press chicken mixture on parchment paper on a cookie sheet. Bake for 12 minutes. Let cool for five minutes.

Top with 1/4 cup of tomato sauce, a handful of low-fat cheese, basil and mushrooms (shiitake). Bake for 6-8 minutes more, or until toppings are melted. Let cool for five minutes. Slice and serve. Alternatively, you may want to try cauliflower crust version:

Grate half of the large cauliflower and steam it for 15 minutes. Squeeze the excess water out and let cool. Mix in 2 eggs, one cup low-fat mozzarella, and salt and pepper. Pat into a 10-inch round on the prepared cookie sheet. Brush with oil and bake until golden. Add the topping as above.

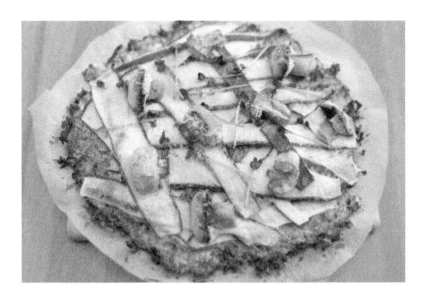

Side dishes

Green Superfoods Rice

Serves: 8

Ingredients - Allergies: SF, GF, DF, EF, V, NF

- 1 cup spinach or any other leafy greens
- 1 cup leeks
- 1/2 cup or more cilantro leaves or parsley
- 1 jalapeno or serrano pepper
- 2 cloves garlic
- 1/4 cup coconut oil
- 1 cup brown rice
- 1 cup quinoa
- 3 tbsp flax seeds meal
- 3 cups water
- 1/2 tsp. salt (more to taste)

Instructions

Pulse the spinach, leeks, cilantro, pepper, and garlic in a food processor. Do it until they become very finely chopped.

Heat the oil in a pot over high heat. Add the rice and quinoa and stir continuously for 5-8 minutes, until the rice is starting to turn light golden brown. Add the water, salt. Cover and boil for 5 minutes. Stir, and lower the heat to simmer for another 10 minutes. Stir in the green paste from the step 1 and cook until the rice is fluffy. Serve with additional salt, cilantro leaves, and lime if desired.

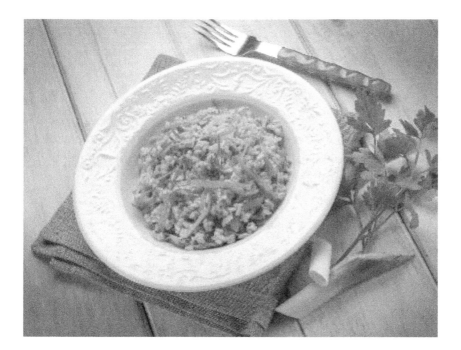

Baked Sweet Potatoes

Serves 2

Ingredients - Allergies: SF, GF, DF, EF, V, NF

• 2 medium sweet potatoes

Instructions

Heat oven to 425 degrees F. Quarter sweet potatoes and place them in a casserole with a lid. Bake until tender when pierced with a fork (40 minutes approx.).

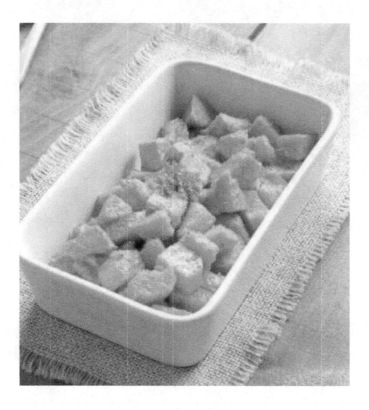

Asparagus with mushrooms and hazelnuts

Serves 4

Ingredients - Allergies: SF, GF, DF, EF, V

- 2 tbsp. lemon juice
- 1/4 tsp sea salt
- 1 pound fresh asparagus, ends trimmed
- 2 tbsp. coconut oil
- 6 cups mushrooms
- 1/2 cup green onions, sliced
- 2 tbsp. hazelnuts, toasted and finely chopped

Instructions

Add the lemon juice, 1 tbsp. of the oil, salt, and pepper in a small bowl. Boil water in a pan and add the asparagus. Boil for few minutes. Heat the remaining 1 tbsp. oil in a pan on high heat. Add mushrooms and cook them until they are soft. Add green onions and sauté 1 more minute. Add the asparagus, and cook another 3 minutes. Remove from the heat and slowly add in the lemon juice mixture. Add the toasted hazelnuts over the top.

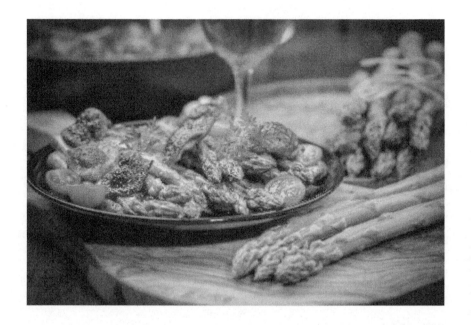

Cauliflower rice side dish

Serves 2

Ingredients - Allergies: SF, GF, DF, EF, V, NF

- 1 head cauliflower
- 2 Tbs coconut oil
- Sea salt, garlic or ginger (optional seasonings)

Instructions

Place the cauliflower into a food processor and pulse it until a grainy rice-like consistency. Season with sea salt. Meanwhile, heat a large sauté pan over high heat. Add coconut oil when hot. Sauté cauliflower in a pan with oil and any additional seasonings if desired.

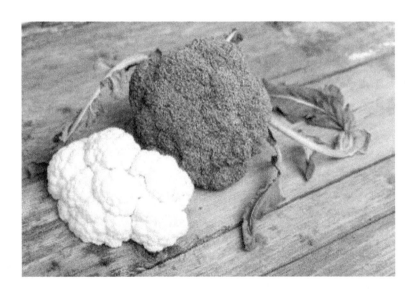

Crockpot

Pork Tenderloin with peppers and onions
Serves 3-4

Ingredients - Allergies: SF, GF, DF, EF, NF

- 1 tbsp. coconut oil
- 1 pound pork loin
- 1 tbsp. caraway seeds
- 1/2 tsp sea salt
- 1 red onion, thinly sliced
- 2 red bell peppers, sliced
- 4 cloves of garlic, minced
- 1/4-1/3 cup chicken broth

Instructions

Wash and chop vegetables. Slice pork loin, and season with caraway seeds and sea salt. Heat a pan over medium heat. Add coconut oil when hot. Add pork loin and brown slightly. Add onions and mushrooms, and continue to sauté until onions are translucent. Add peppers, garlic and chicken broth. Simmer until vegetables are tender and pork is fully cooked.

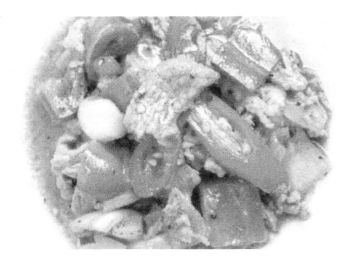

Beef Bourguinon

Serves 8-10

Ingredients - Allergies: SF, GF, DF, EF

- 4 pounds cubed lean beef
- 1 cup red wine
- 1/3 cup coconut oil
- 1 tsp. thyme
- 2 cloves garlic, crushed
- 1 onion, diced
- 1 pound mushrooms, sliced
- 1/3 cup almond flour

Instructions

Marinate beef in wine, oil, thyme and pepper for few hours at room temperature or 6-8 hours in the fridge. Cook garlic and onion in a pan until soft. Add mushrooms. Cook until they are browned. Drain beef liquid. Place beef in slow cooker. Sprinkle flour over the beef and stir to coat. Add mushroom mixture on top. Pour reserved marinade over all. Cook on low for 7-9 hrs.

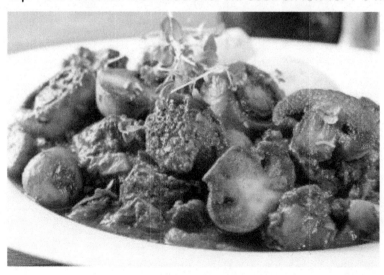

Italian Chicken

Serves 6-8

Ingredients - Allergies: SF, GF, DF, EF

- 1 skinless chicken, cut into pieces
- 1/4 cup almond flour
- 1 1/2 tsp. salt
- 1/8 tsp. pepper
- 1/2 cup chicken broth
- 1 cup sliced mushrooms
- 1/2 tsp. paprika
- 1 zucchini, sliced into medium pieces
- parsley to garnish

Instructions

Season chicken with 1 tsp. salt. Combine flour, pepper, remaining salt, and paprika. Coat chicken pieces with this mixture. Place zucchini first in a crockpot. Pour broth over zucchini. Arrange chicken on top. Cover and cook on low for 6 to 8 hours or until tender. Turn control to high, add mushrooms, cover, and cook on high for additional 10-15 minutes. Garnish with parsley.

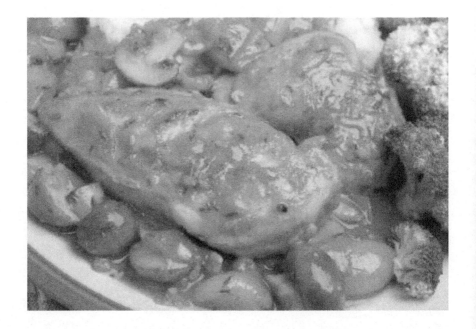

Ropa Vieja

Ingredients - Allergies: SF, GF, DF, EF, NF

6 servings

- 1 tbsp. coconut oil
- 2 pounds beef flank steak
- 1 cup beef broth
- 1 cup tomato sauce
- 1 small onion, sliced
- 1 green bell pepper sliced into strips
- 2 cloves garlic, chopped
- 1/2 cup tomato paste
- 1 tsp. ground cumin
- 1 tsp. chopped cilantro
- 1 tbsp. olive oil & 1 tbsp. lemon juice

Instructions

Heat oil in a skillet over high heat. Brown the flank steak on each side (4 minutes per side). Move the beef to a slow cooker. Add in the beef broth and tomato sauce, then add the onion, bell pepper, garlic , tomato paste , cumin, cilantro, olive oil and lemon juice. Stir until blended. Cover, and cook on high for 4 hours, or on Low for up to 8 hours. When ready to serve, shred meat and serve with brown rice or quinoa and salad.

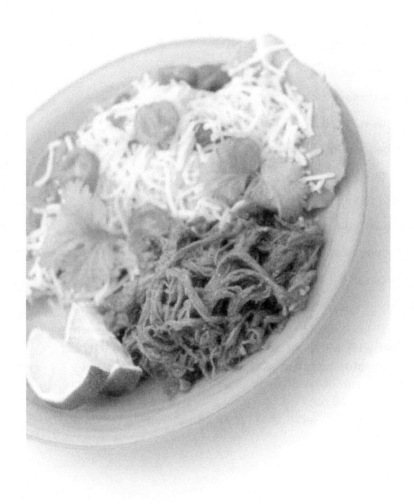

Lemon Roast Chicken

Serves 6-8

Ingredients - Allergies: SF, GF, DF, EF, NF

- 1 whole skinless chicken
- 1 dash Salt
- 1 dash Pepper
- 1 tsp. Oregano
- 2 cloves minced garlic
- 2 tbsp. coconut oil
- 1/4 cup Water
- 3 tbsp. Lemon juice

- Rosemary

Instructions

Wash chicken and season with salt and pepper. Sprinkle half of oregano and garlic inside chicken cavity. Add coconut oil to a frying pan. Brown chicken on all sides and transfer to crock pot. Sprinkle with oregano and garlic. Add water to fry pan and stir to loosen brown bits. Pour into crock pot and cover. Cook on low 7 hours. Add lemon juice when cooking is done. Transfer chicken to cutting board and carve chicken. Skim fat. Pour juice into sauce bowl. Serve with rosemary and some juice over chicken.

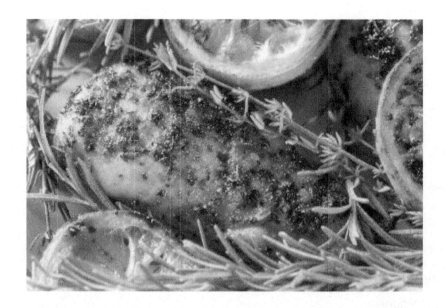

Slow cooker pork loin

Serves 4-6

Ingredients - Allergies: SF, GF, DF, EF, NF

- 1-1/2 lb pork loin
- 1 cup tomato sauce
- 2 zucchinis, sliced
- 1 head cauliflower, separated into medium florets
- 1-2 Tbs dried basil
- 1/2 tsp sea salt (optional)

Instructions

   Add all of the ingredients to a crock pot.

   Cook on high for 3-4 hours or low 7-8 hours.

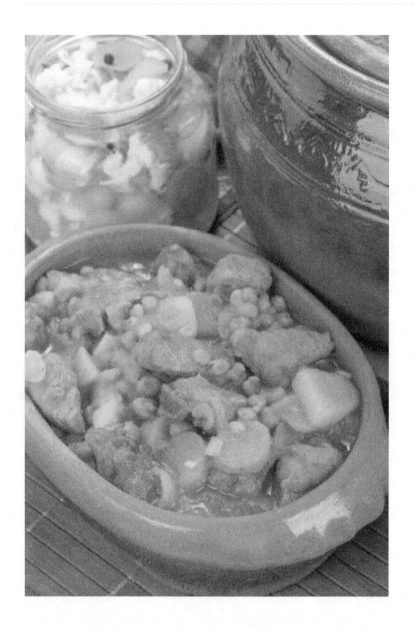

Flounder with Orange Coconut Oil
Serves 6

Ingredients - Allergies: SF, GF, DF, EF, NF

- 31/2 lbs. flounder
- 3 tbsp. white wine
- 3 tbsp. lemon juice
- 3 tbsp. coconut oil
- 3 tbsp. parsley
- 2 tbsp. orange zest
- 1/2 tsp. salt
- 1/2 cup chopped scallions

Instructions

Preheat oven to 325F. Sprinkle fish with pepper and salt.
Place fish in the baking dish. Sprinkle orange zest on top of the fish. Melt remaining coconut oil and add the parsley and scallions to the coconut oil and pour over flounder. Then add in the white wine.
Place in oven and bake for 15 minutes. Serve fish with extra juice on a side.

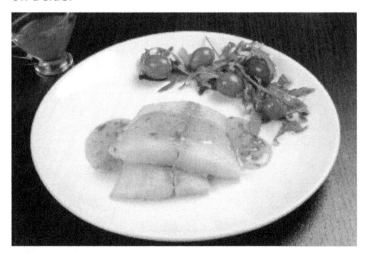

Grilled Salmon

Serves 4

Ingredients - Allergies: SF, GF, DF, EF, NF

- 4 (4 ounce) filets salmon
- 1/4 cup coconut oil
- 2 tbsp. fish sauce
- 2 tbsp. lemon juice
- 2 tbsp. thinly sliced green onion
- 1 clove garlic, minced & 3/4 tsp. ground ginger
- 1/2 tsp. crushed red pepper flakes
- 1/2 tsp. sesame oil
- 1/8 tsp. salt

Instructions

Whisk together coconut oil, fish sauce, garlic, ginger, red chili flakes, lemon juice, green onions, sesame oil, and salt. Put fish in a glass dish, and pour marinade over. Cover and refrigerate for 4 hours.
Preheat grill. Place salmon on grill. Grill until fish becomes tender. Turn halfway during cooking.

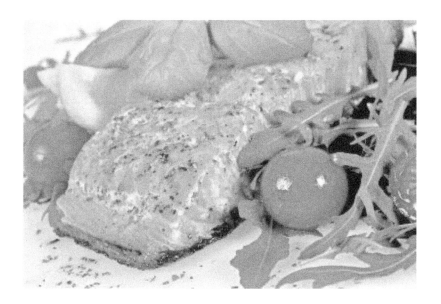

Crab Cakes

Serves 6-8

Ingredients - Allergies: SF, GF, DF, NF

- 3 lbs. crabmeat
- 3 beaten eggs
- 3 cups <u>flax</u> seeds meal
- 3 tbsp. mustard
- 2 tbsp. grated horseradish
- 1/2 cup <u>coconut</u> oil
- 1 tsp. lemon rind
- 3 tbsp. lemon juice
- 2 tbsp. parsley
- 1/2 tsp. cayenne pepper
- 2 tsp. fish sauce

Instructions

In medium bowl combine all ingredients except oil. Shape in to smallish hamburgers. In fry pan heat oil and cook patties for 3-4 minutes on each side or until golden brown. Optionally, bake them in the oven.

Serve as appetizers or as main course with large fiber salad.

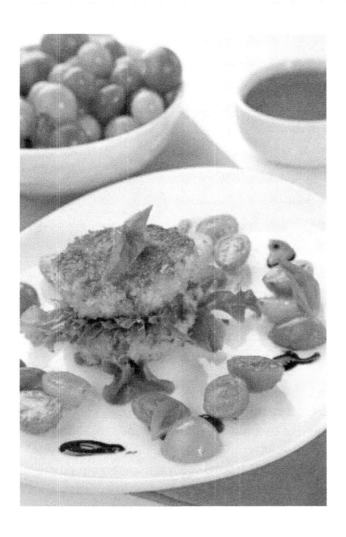

Sweets

Sweet Superfoods pie crust

Ingredients - Allergies: SF, GF, DF

- 11/3 cups blanched <u>almond</u> flour
- 1/3 cup tapioca flour
- 1/2 tsp. sea salt
- 1 large egg
- 1/4 cup <u>coconut</u> oil
- 2 tbsp. coconut sugar or raw <u>honey</u>
- 1 tsp of ground <u>vanilla</u> bean

Instructions

Place almond flour, tapioca flour, sea salt, vanilla, egg and coconut sugar (if you use coconut sugar) in the bowl of a food processor. Process 2-3 times to combine. Add oil and raw honey (if you use raw honey) and pulse with several one-second pulses and then let the food processor run until the mixture comes together. Pour dough onto a sheet of plastic wrap. Wrap and then press the dough into a 9-inch disk. Refrigerate for 30 minutes.

Remove plastic wrap. Press dough onto the bottom and up the sides of a 9-inch buttered pie dish. Crimp a little bit the edges of crust. Cool in the refrigerator for 20 minutes. Put the oven rack to middle position and preheat oven to 375F. Put in the oven and bake until golden brown.

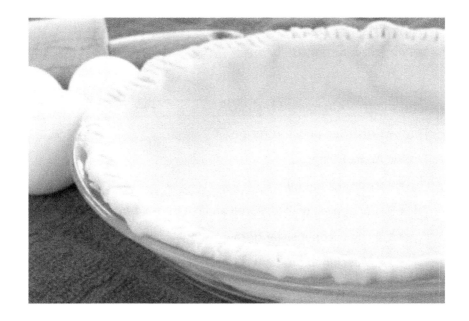

Apple Pie

Serving Size: Serves 8

Ingredients - Allergies: SF, GF, DF

For the Crust: See previous recipe

For the Apple Filling:

- 2 tbsp. coconut oil
- 9 sour apples, peeled, cored and cut into 1/4-inch thick slices
- 1/4 cup coconut sugar or raw honey
- 1/2 tsp. cinnamon
- 1/8 tsp. sea salt
- 1/2 cup coconut milk

For the Topping:

- 1 cup ground nuts and seeds

Instructions

Filling: Melt coconut oil in a large pot over medium heat. Add apples, coconut sugar or raw honey, cinnamon and sea salt. Increase heat to medium-high and cook, stirring occasionally, until apples release their moisture and sugar is melted. Pour coconut milk or cream over apples and continue to cook until apples are soft and liquid has thickened, about 5 minutes, stirring occasionally.

Pour the filling into the crust and then top with topping. Place a pie shield over the edges of the crust to avoid burning. Bake until topping is just turning golden brown. Cool and serve.

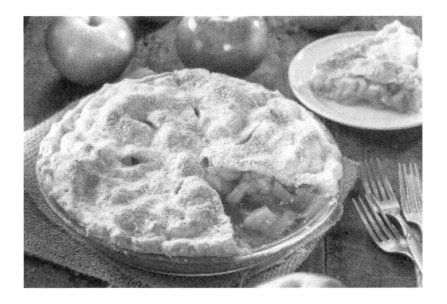

Superfoods Dark Chocolate

Instructions - Allergies: SF, GF, DF, EF, V, NF

Mix 1/4 cup of coconut oil with 1/4 to 1/2 cup of cocoa powder (unsweetened, ideally organic and unprocessed) and some raw honey to taste. You really should experiment with cocoa and honey amount. Maybe start with equal amount of coconut oil, cocoa and honey, mix it and then increase amount of cocoa to your taste. Form balls or put in the ice cube tray. Put it in the fridge and 1 hour later you'll have great homemade Superfoods chocolate!

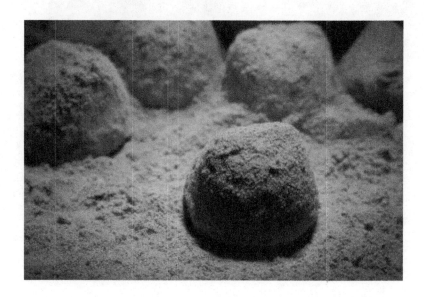

Fruits dipped in Superfoods chocolate

Ingredients - Allergies: SF, GF, DF, EF, V

- 2 apples or 2 bananas or a bowl of strawberries or any fruit that can be dipped in melted chocolate
- 1/2 cup of melted superfoods chocolate (see earlier recipe)
- 2 tbsp. chopped nuts (almond, walnut, Brazil nuts) or seeds (hemp, chia, sesame, flax seeds meal)

Instructions

Cut apple in wedges or cut banana in quarters. Melt the chocolate and chop the nuts. Dip fruit in chocolate, sprinkle with nuts or seeds and lay on tray. Transfer the tray to the fridge so the chocolate can harden; serve. If you don't want chocolate, cover fruits with almond or sunflower butter and sprinkle with chia or hemp seeds and cut it into chunks and serve.

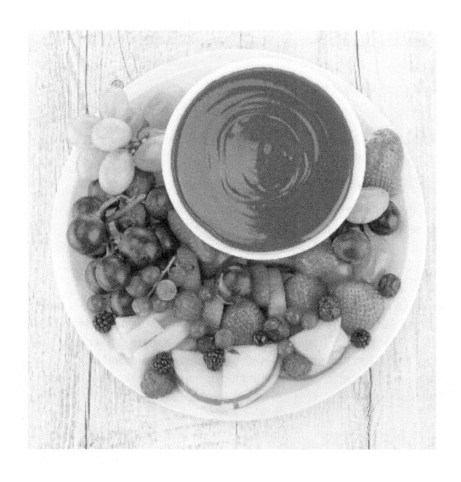

Superfoods No-Bake Cookies

Ingredients - Allergies: SF, GF, DF, EF, V

- 1/2 cup coconut milk

- 1/2 cup cocoa powder

- 1/2 cup coconut oil

- 1/2 cup raw honey

- 2 cups finely shredded coconut

- 1 cup large flake coconut

- 2 tsp of ground vanilla bean

- 1/2 cup chopped almonds or chia seeds (optional)

- 1/2 cup almond butter (optional)

Instructions

Combine the coconut milk, coconut oil and cacao powder in a saucepan. Cook the coconut mixture over medium heat, stirring until it comes to a boil and then boil for 1 minute. Remove the mixture from the heat and stir in the shredded coconut, large flake coconut, raw honey and the vanilla. Add additional ingredients if you want. Spoon the mixture to a parchment lined baking sheet to cool.

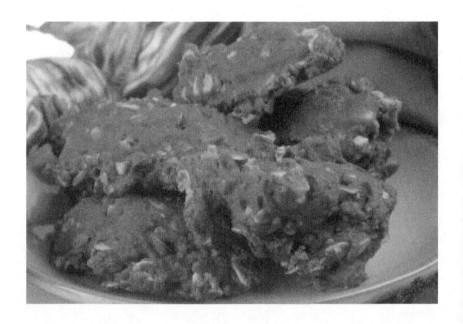

Raw Brownies

Ingredients - Allergies: SF, GF, DF, EF, V

- 1 1/2 cups walnuts
- 1 cup pitted dates
- 1 1/2 tsp. ground vanilla bean
- 1/3 cup unsweetened cocoa powder
- 1/3 cup almond butter

Instructions

Add walnuts and salt to a food processor or blender. Mix until finely ground.

Add the vanilla, dates, and cocoa powder to the blender. Mix well and optionally add a couple drops of water at a time to make the mixture stick together.

Transfer the mixture into a pan and top with almond butter.

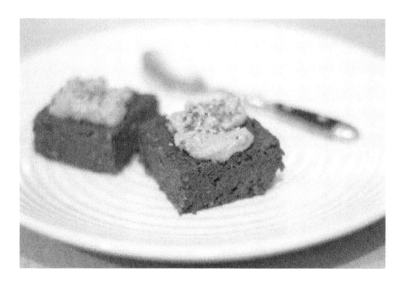

Superfoods Ice cream

Allergies: SF, GF, DF, EF, V, NF

Freeze a banana cut into chunks and process it in blender once frozen and add half a tsp. of cinnamon or 1 tsp. of cocoa or both and eat it as ice-cream.

Other option would be to add one spoon of almond butter and mix it with mashed banana, it's also a delicious ice cream.

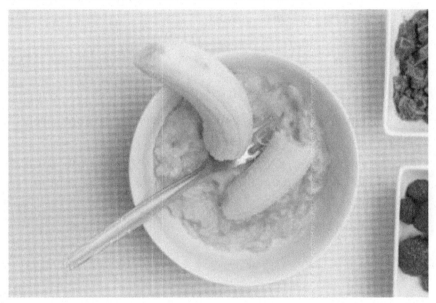

Apple Spice Cookies

Ingredients - Allergies: SF, GF, DF, EF, V

- 1 cup unsweetened <u>almond</u> butter
- 1/2 cup raw <u>honey</u>
- 1 egg & 1/2 tsp salt
- 1 apple, diced
- 1 tsp cinnamon
- 1/4 tsp ground cloves
- 1/8 tsp nutmeg
- 1 tsp fresh ginger, grated

Instructions

Heat oven to 350 degrees F. Combine almond butter, egg, raw honey and salt in a bowl. Add apple, spices, and ginger and stir. Spoon batter onto a baking sheet 1 inches apart. Bake until set. Remove cookies and allow to cool on a cooling rack.

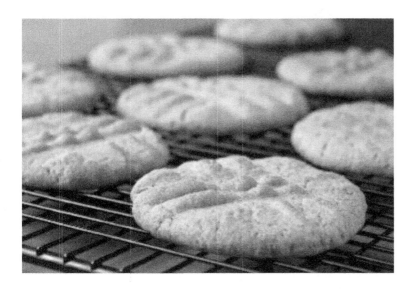

Superfoods Macaroons

Ingredients - Allergies: SF, GF, DF, NF

- 3 egg whites

- 1/2 cup coconut sugar

- 1/4 tsp. salt

- 1 cup unsweetened flaked coconut

- 1/2 cup soft dried apricots, coarsely chopped (3 ounces)

Heat the oven to 325 degrees. Whisk together egg whites, sugar, and salt in a bowl until frothy. Add apricots and coconut and mix to combine.

Shape mixture into mounds with hands and place one inch apart on baking sheet.

Bake until lightly golden, 35 to 40 minutes. Rotate sheet halfway through. You can cover them with Superfoods Dark Chocolate.

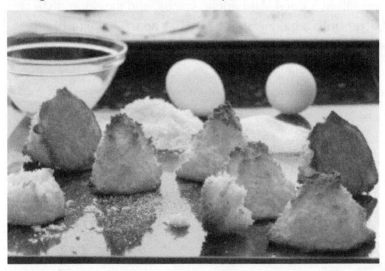

Superfoods Stuffed Apples

Allergies: SF, GF, DF, EF, V

Core 10 apples, fill them with Superfoods No Bake Balls mix and bake them in the oven for 25-30 minutes.

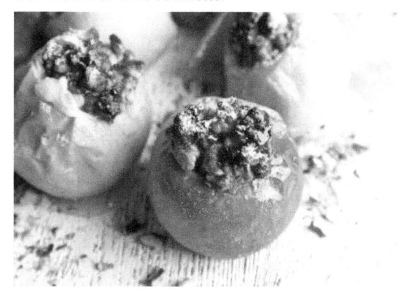

Whipped Coconut cream

Ingredients - Allergies: SF, GF, DF, EF, V, NF

- 4 cups of any fresh berries
- 2 lemons
- 1 can full fat coconut milk (14 oz.), refrigerated overnight
- 1 tsp of ground vanilla bean
- 2 Tbsp. raw honey
- Dash of cardamom, nutmeg and clove (optional)

Instructions

Separate coconut cream from the milk by putting it overnight in the fridge. Don't shake it before opening.

Open the can of coconut milk and scrape out the cream into a bowl. Use the saved milk for smoothies or other recipes.

Add cardamom, raw honey and vanilla. Whip the cream with a hand mixer until fluffy. Put in the fridge.

Wash berries and place in serving bowls or glasses. Squeeze the lemon over the berries. Place a big scoop of cream on top of the berries and serve.

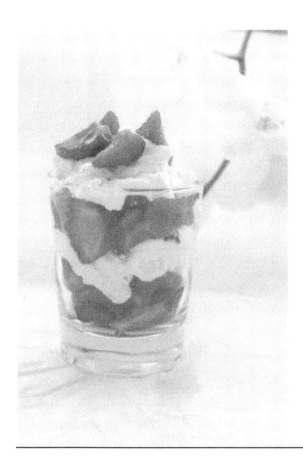

Granola Mix

Ingredients - Allergies: SF, GF, DF, EF, V

- 10 Cup Rolled Oats
- 1/2 Pound Shredded Coconut
- 2 Cup Raw Sunflower Seeds
- 1 Cup Sesame Seeds or chia seeds
- 3 Cup Chopped Nuts
- 1-1/2 Cup -Water
- 1-1/2 Cup coconut oil
- 1 Cup raw honey
- 1-1/2 Tsp. Salt
- 2 Tsp. Cinnamon
- 1 tbsp. of ground vanilla bean

- Dried cranberries

Instructions

Turn the oven on and heat oven to 300F. Combine oats, coconut, sunflower seeds, sesame seed, cranberries and nuts (can include almonds, pecans, walnuts, or a combination of all of them). Blend well.
Combine water, oil, raw honey, salt, cinnamon and vanilla in a large pan. Heat until raw honey is dissolved, but don't boil.
Pour the honey over the dry ingredients and stir well. Spread onto cookie sheets. Bake 25 to 30 minutes, and stir occasionally. Let it cool. Store in a cool dry place.

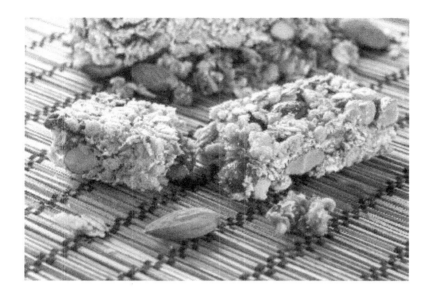

Pumpkin pie

Ingredients - Allergies: SF, GF, DF, NF

- 11/2 cup homemade pumpkin puree
- 3 eggs
- 1/2 cup coconut milk
- 1/2 cup raw <u>honey</u>
- 1 tbsp. ground cinnamon
- 1 tsp. nutmeg
- ⅛ tsp. sea salt
- 1 Superfoods Sweet Pie Crust, unbaked

Instructions

In a food processor combine pumpkin puree, and eggs. Pulse in cinnamon, nutmeg, coconut milk, raw honey, and salt. Pour filling into Superfoods Sweet Pie Crust and bake at 350° for 45 minutes. Allow the pie to cool and then refrigerate for 2 hours.

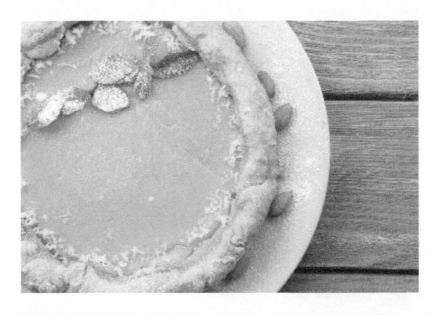

Blueberry Cream Pie

Ingredients - Allergies: SF, GF, DF, EF, V, NF

- Sweet Superfoods pie crust

  Filling:

- 2 Teaspoons plant-based gelatin, dissolved in 2 Tbsp. hot water

- 1/3 cup lemon juice

- 1/3 cup raw honey

- 1 can coconut milk, chilled

- 4 cups blueberries for serving

Instructions

Mix the gelatin and water together. Stir to dissolve and add the lemon juice. Whip coconut milk and raw honey with electric mixer about 15 minutes. Add the gelatin liquid to the whipped cream. Pour the filling into the crust. Filling will set up in the refrigerator.

Chill for at 4 hours until set, and serve with lots of berries.

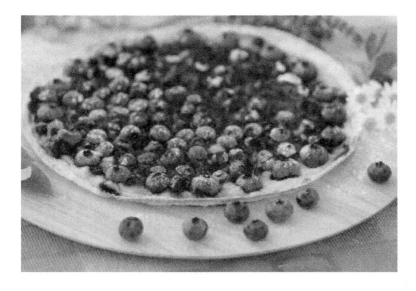

Upside down Apple Cake

Ingredients - Allergies: SF, GF, DF

Bottom Fruit Layer:

- 2 tbsp. coconut oil, melted
- 1 apple, sliced, or 1/4 cup blueberries, plums, banana etc.
- 2 tbsp. walnut chunks
- 2 tbsp. coconut sugar
- 1 tsp ground cinnamon.

Top Cake Layer:

- 2 eggs, beaten.
- 1/3 cup raw honey
- 1/4 cup unsweetened coconut milk, or unsweetened almond milk.
- 1 tsp ground vanilla bean
- 1 tsp lemon juice.
- 1 banana, mashed, or 1/4 cup blueberries
- 1/3 cup coconut flour

Instructions

Heat the oven (350 F), and grease a 9 inch cake pan.

Place 2 tbsps. coconut oil into cake pan, and put pan into preheating oven for a couple minutes to melt oil. Make sure oil is evenly distributed all over the bottom of the pan.

Sprinkle 2 tbsps. coconut sugar all over the oil.

Sprinkle 1 tsp cinnamon on top of sweetened layer.

Layer apple slices or blueberries on top of sweetened layer. Add optional walnut pieces to fruit layer. Set aside.

Combine all the "top cake layer" ingredients in a large mixing bowl except for the coconut flour. Mix and add the coconut flour and mix well.

Spoon batter on top of fruit layer and spread evenly.

Bake until center is set.

Remove from oven and let cool.

Slide a butter knife between cake and edge of pan to loosen cake. Turn cake pan upside down onto a large plate or serving platter. Cake should fall onto plate. If not, use spatula to take the cake out.

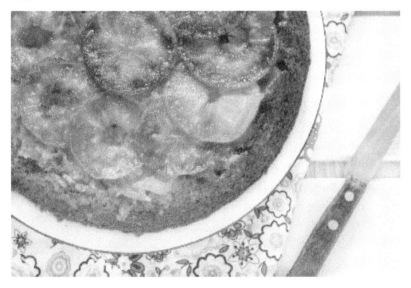

Raw Vegan Reese's Cups

"Peanut" Butter Filling

- 1/2 cup sunflower seeds butter
- 1/2 cup almond butter
- 1 Tbsp. raw honey
- 2 Tbsp. melted coconut oil

Superfoods Chocolate Part:

- 1/2 cup cacao powder
- 2 Tbsp. raw honey
- 1/3 cup coconut oil (melted)

Instructions

Mix the "Peanut" butter filling ingredients. Put a spoonful of the mixture into each muffin cup.

Refrigerate. Mix Superfoods chocolate ingredients. Put a spoonful of the Superfoods chocolate mixture over the "peanut" butter mixture. Freeze!

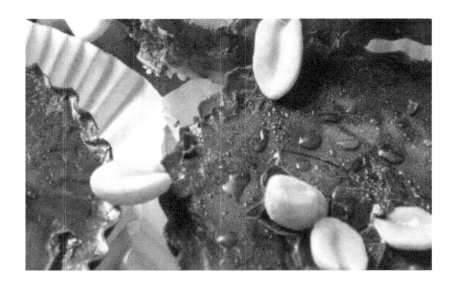

Raw Vegan Coffee Cashew Cream Cake

Coffee Cashew Cream

- 2 cups raw cashews
- 1 tsp. of ground <u>vanilla</u> bean
- 3 tablespoons melted <u>coconut</u> oil
- 1/4 cup raw <u>honey</u>
- 1/3 cup very strong coffee or triple espresso shot

Crust

See recipe for Raw Walnuts Pie Crust

Instructions

Blend all ingredients for the cream, pour it onto the crust and refrigerate. Garnish with coffee beans.

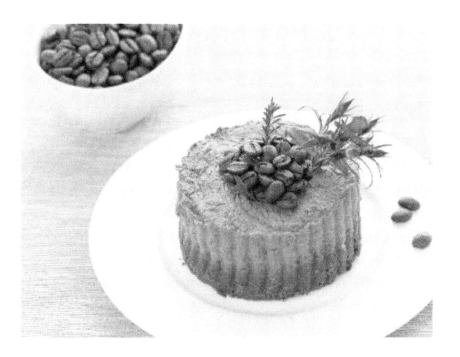

Raw Vegan Chocolate Cashew Truffles

Ingredients

- 1 cup ground cashews
- 1 tsp. of ground vanilla bean
- 1/2 cup coconut oil
- 1/4 cup raw honey
- 2 tbsp. flax seeds meal
- 2 tbsp. hemp hearts
- 2 tbsp. cacao powder

Instructions

Mix all ingredients and make truffles. Sprinkle coconut flakes on top.

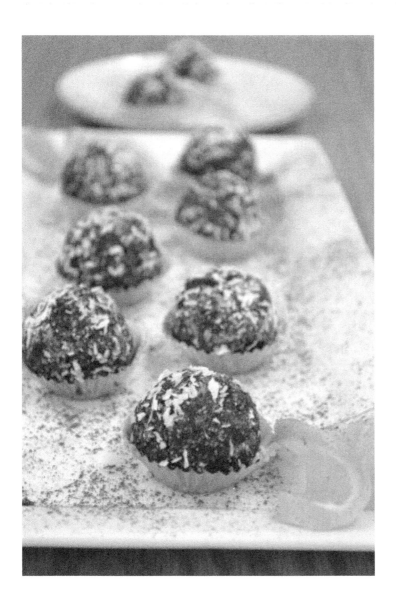

Raw Vegan Double Almond Raw Chocolate Tart

Ingredients

- 1½ cups raw almonds
- ¼ cup coconut oil, melted
- 1 tablespoon raw honey or royal jelly
- 8 ounces dark chocolate, chopped
- 1 cup coconut milk
- 1/2 cup unsweetened shredded coconut

Instructions

Crust

Ground almonds and add melted coconut oil, raw honey and combine. Using a spatula, spread this mixture into the tart or pie pan.

Filling

Put chopped chocolate in a bowl, heat coconut milk and pour over chocolate and whisk together. Pour filling into tart shell. Refrigerate. Toast almond slivers chips and sprinkle over tart.

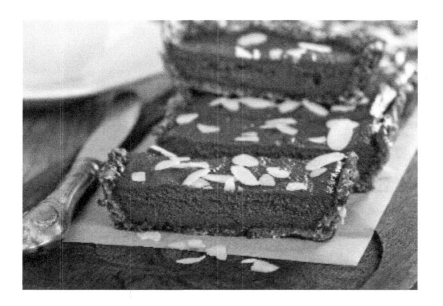

Raw Vegan Bounty Bars

"Peanut" Butter Filling

- 2 cups desiccated coconut
- 3 Tbsp. coconut oil - melted
- 1 cup coconut cream - full fat
- 4 Tbsp. of raw honey
- 1 Tsp. ground vanilla bean
- pinch of sea salt

Superfoods Chocolate Part:

- 1/2 cup cacao powder
- 2 Tbsp. raw honey
- 1/3 cup coconut oil (melted)

Instructions

Mix coconut oil, coconut cream, honey, vanilla and salt. Pour over desiccated coconut and mix well. Mold coconut mixture into balls, small bars similar to bounty and freeze. Or pour whole mixture into a tray, freeze and cut into small bars.

Make Superfoods Chocolate mixture, warm it up and dip frozen coconut into chocolate and put on a tray and freeze again.

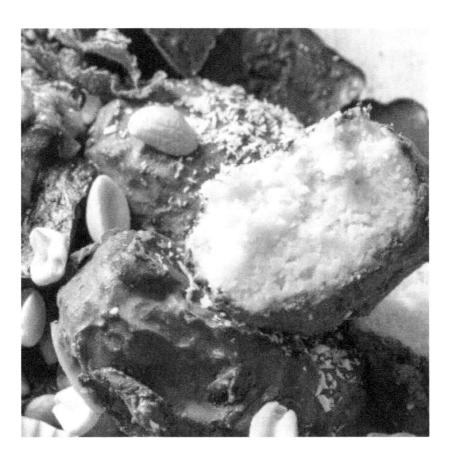

Raw Vegan Tartlets with Coconut Cream

Crust:

See recipe for Raw Walnuts Pie Crust. Make tartlets.

Pudding:

• 1 avocado

• 2 tablespoons coconut oil

• 2 tablespoons raw honey

• 2 tablespoons cacao powder

• 1 teaspoon ground vanilla bean

• Pinch of salt

• 1/4 cup Almond milk, as needed

Coconut cream:

See recipe for "Whipped Coconut Cream". Add 1/2 tsp. cinnamon and whip again.

To make the pudding: blend all the ingredients in the food processor until smooth and thick. Spread evenly into tartlet crusts. Optionally, put some goji berries on top of the pudding layer.

Make the coconut cream, spread it on top of the pudding layer, and put back in the fridge overnight. Serve with one blueberry on top of each tartlet.

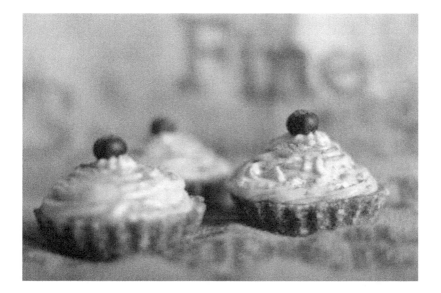

Raw Vegan "Peanut" Butter Truffles

Ingredients

- 5 tbsp. sunflower seed butter
- 1 tbsp. coconut oil
- 1 tbsp. raw honey
- 1 teaspoons ground vanilla bean
- 3/4 cup almond flour
- 1 tbsp. flax seeds meal
- pinch of salt
- 1 tbsp. cacao butter
- hemp hearts (optional)
- 1/4 cup Superfoods Chocolate

Instructions

Add sunflower seed butter, coconut oil, raw honey, vanilla, almond flour, flaxseed meal and salt to a large bowl.

Mix until all ingredients are incorporated.

Roll the dough into 1-inch balls, place them on parchment paper and refrigerate for half an hour (yield about 14 truffles)

Dip each truffle in the melted Superfoods Chocolate, one at the time, and place them back on the pan with parchment paper or coat them in cocoa powder or coconut flakes.

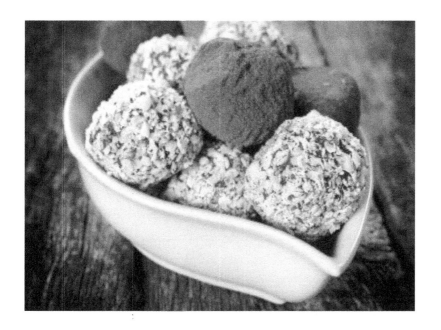

Raw Vegan Chocolate Pie

Crust

- 2 cups almonds, soaked overnight and drained
- 1 cup pitted dates, soaked overnight and drained
- 1 cup chopped dried apricots
- 1 1/2 tsp. ground vanilla bean
- 2 tsp. chia seeds
- 1 banana

Filling

- 4 Tbsp. raw cacao powder
- 3 Tbsp. raw honey
- 2 ripe avocados
- 2 Tbsp. organic coconut oil
- 2 Tbsp. almond milk (if needed, check for consistency first)

Instructions

Add almonds and banana to a food processor or blender. Mix until it forms a thick ball. Add the vanilla, dates, and apricot chunks to the blender. Mix well and optionally add a couple drops of water at a time to make the mixture stick together.

Spread in a 10 inch dis.

Mix filling ingredients in a blender and add almond milk if necessary. Add filling to the crust and refrigerate.

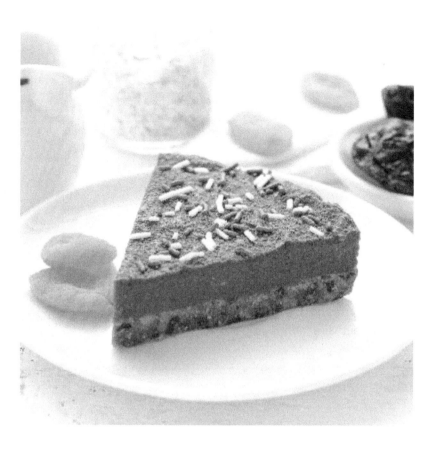

Raw Vegan Chocolate Walnut Truffles

Ingredients

- 1 cup ground walnuts
- 1 tsp. cinnamon
- 1/2 cup coconut oil
- 1/4 cup raw honey
- 2 tbsp. chia seeds
- 2 tbsp. cacao powder

Instructions

Mix all ingredients and make truffles. Coat with cinnamon, coconut flakes or chopped almonds.

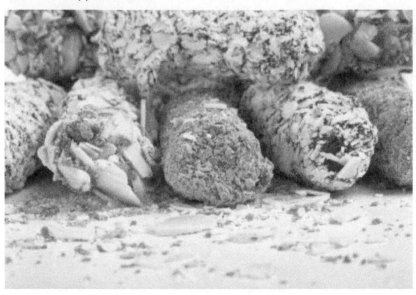

Superfoods Reference Book

Unfortunately, I had to take out the whole Superfoods Reference Book out of all of my books because parts of that book are featured on my blog. I joined Kindle Direct Publishing Select program which allows me to have all my books free for 5 days every 3 months. Unfortunately, KDP Select program also means that all my books have to have unique content that is not available in any other online store or on the Internet (including my blog). I didn't want to remove parts of Superfoods Reference book that is already on my blog because I want that all people have free access to that information. I also wanted to be part of KDP Select program because that is an option to give my book for free to anyone. So, some sections of my Superfoods Reference Book can be found on my blog, under Superfoods menu on my blog. Complete Reference book is available for subscribers to my Superfoods Today Newsletter. Subscribers to my Newsletter will also get information whenever any of my books becomes free on Amazon. I will not offer any product pitches or anything similar to my subscribers, only Superfoods related information, recipes and weight loss and fitness tips. So, subscribe to my newsletter, download Superfoods Today Desserts free eBook which has complete Superfood Reference book included and have the opportunity to get all of my future books for free.

REFERENCES:

Morelli SA1, Torre JB, Eisenberger NI. The neural bases of feeling understood and not understood. Soc Cogn Affect Neurosci. 2014 Feb 14. [Epub ahead of print]

Oschman JL. Can electrons act as antioxidants? A review and commentary. J Altern Complement Med. 2007 Nov;13(9):955-67.

Ye L1, Guo J1, Ge RS2. Environmental pollutants and hydroxysteroid dehydrogenases. Vitam Horm. 2014;94:349-90. doi: 10.1016/B978-0-12-800095-3.00013-4.

Albuquerque TG1, Costa HS, Sanches-Silva A, Santos M, Trichopoulou A, D'Antuono F, Alexieva I, Boyko N, Costea C, Fedosova K, Karpenko D, Kilasonia Z, Koçaoglu B, Finglas P. Traditional foods from the Black Sea region as a potential source of minerals. J Sci Food Agric. 2013 Nov;93(14):3535-44. doi: 10.1002/jsfa.6164. Epub 2013 May 10.

Ali M1, Thomson M, Afzal M. Garlic and onions: their effect on eicosanoid metabolism and its clinical relevance. Prostaglandins Leukot Essent Fatty Acids. 2000 Feb;62(2):55-73.

Bornhoeft J1, Castaneda D, Nemoseck T, Wang P, Henning SM, Hong MY. The protective effects of green tea polyphenols: lipid profile, inflammation, and antioxidant capacity in rats fed an atherogenic diet and dextran sodium sulfate. J Med Food. 2012 Aug;15(8):726-32. doi: 10.1089/jmf.2011.0258. Epub 2012 Jun 25.

Ceylon Med J. 2014 Mar;59(1):4-8. doi: 10.4038/cmj.v59i1.6731.

Senadheera SP1, Ekanayake S, Wanigatunge C. Antioxidant potential of green leafy porridges.

Gülçin İ. Antioxidant activity of food constituents: an overview. Arch Toxicol. 2012 Mar;86(3):345-91. doi: 10.1007/s00204-011-0774-2. Epub 2011 Nov 20.

Heim KC1, Angers P, Léonhart S, Ritz BW. Anti-inflammatory and neuroactive properties of selected fruit extracts. J Med Food. 2012 Sep;15(9):851-4. doi: 10.1089/jmf.2011.0265. Epub 2012 Aug 7.

Meral O1, Alpay M, Kismali G, Kosova F, Cakir DU, Pekcan M, Yigit S, Sel T. Capsaicin inhibits cell proliferation by cytochrome c release in gastric cancer cells. Tumour Biol. 2014 Mar 30.

Moon JK1, Shibamoto T. Antioxidant assays for plant and food components. J Agric Food Chem. 2009 Mar 11;57(5):1655-66. doi: 10.1021/jf803537k.

Nagaraja P1, Aradhana N, Suma A, Shivakumar A, Chamaraja NA. Quantification of antioxidants by using chlorpromazine hydrochloride: application of the method to food and medicinal plant samples. Anal Sci. 2014;30(2):251-6.

Johnston C. Functional Foods as Modifiers of Cardiovascular Disease. Am J Lifestyle Med. 2009 Jul;3(1 Suppl):39S-43S.

Hernández-Ortega M1, Ortiz-Moreno A, Hernández-Navarro MD, Chamorro-Cevallos G, Dorantes-Alvarez L, Necoechea-Mondragón H. Antioxidant, antinociceptive, and anti-inflammatory effects of carotenoids extracted from dried pepper (Capsicum annuum L.). J Biomed Biotechnol. 2012;2012:524019. doi: 10.1155/2012/524019. Epub 2012 Oct 2.

Nicod N1, Chiva-Blanch G, Giordano E, Dávalos A, Parker RS, Visioli F. Green Tea, Cocoa, and Red Wine Polyphenols Moderately Modulate Intestinal Inflammation and Do Not Increase High-Density Lipoprotein (HDL) Production. J Agric Food Chem. 2014 Mar 12;62(10):2228-32. doi: 10.1021/jf500348u. Epub 2014 Mar 4.

Ownby SL, Fortuno LV, Au AY, Grzanna MW, Rashmir-Raven AM, Frondoza CG. (2014). Expression of pro-inflammatory mediators is inhibited by an avocado/soybean unsaponifiables and epigallocatechin gallate combination. J Inflamm (Lond). 2014 Mar 28;11(1):8.

Pastrana-Bonilla E1, Akoh CC, Sellappan S, Krewer G. Phenolic content and antioxidant capacity of muscadine grapes. J Agric Food Chem. 2003 Aug 27;51(18):5497-503.

Podsędek A1, Redzynia M1, Klewicka E2, Koziołkiewicz M1. Matrix effects on the stability and antioxidant activity of red cabbage anthocyanins under simulated gastrointestinal digestion. Biomed Res Int. 2014;2014:365738. doi: 10.1155/2014/365738. Epub 2014 Jan 19.

Seeram NP. Berry fruits: compositional elements, biochemical activities, and the impact of their intake on human health, performance, and disease. J Agric Food Chem. 2008 Feb 13;56(3):627-9. doi: 10.1021/jf071988k. Epub 2008 Jan 23.

Seeram NP1, Adams LS, Zhang Y, Lee R, Sand D, Scheuller HS, Heber D. Blackberry, black raspberry, blueberry, cranberry, red raspberry, and strawberry extracts inhibit growth and stimulate apoptosis of human cancer cells in vitro. J Agric Food Chem. 2006 Dec 13;54(25):9329-39.

Sharmin H1, Nazma S, Mohiduzzaman M, Cadi PB. Antioxidant capacity and total phenol content of commonly consumed selected vegetables of Bangladesh. Malays J Nutr. 2011 Dec;17(3):377-83.

Thomson SJ1, Rippon P, Butts C, Olsen S, Shaw M, Joyce NI, Eady CC. Inhibition of platelet activation by lachrymatory factor synthase (LFS)-silenced (tearless) onion juice.J Agric Food Chem. 2013 Nov 6;61(44):10574-81. doi: 10.1021/jf4030213. Epub 2013 Oct 22.

Your Free Gift

As a way of saying thanks for your purchase, I'm offering you my FREE eBook that is exclusive to my book and blog readers.

Superfoods Cookbook Book Two has over 70 Superfoods recipes and complements Superfoods Cookbook Book One and it contains Superfoods Salads, Superfoods Smoothies and Superfoods Deserts with ultra-healthy non-refined ingredients. All ingredients are 100% Superfoods.

It also contains Superfoods Reference book which is organized by Superfoods (more than 60 of them, with the list of their benefits), Superfoods spices, all vitamins, minerals and antioxidants. Superfoods Reference Book lists Superfoods that can help with 12 diseases and 9 types of cancer.

http://www.SuperfoodsToday.com/FREE

Other Books from this Author

Superfoods Today Diet is a Kindle Superfoods Diet <u>book</u> that gives you 4 week Superfoods Diet meal plan as well as 2 weeks maintenance meal plan and recipes for weight loss success. It is an extension of Detox book and it's written for people who want to switch to Superfoods lifestyle.

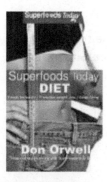

Superfoods Today Body Care is a Kindle <u>book</u> with over 50 Natural Recipes for beautiful skin and hair. It has body scrubs, facial masks and hair care recipes made with the best Superfoods like avocado honey, coconut, olive oil, oatmeal, yogurt, banana and Superfoods herbs like lavender, rosemary, mint, sage, hibiscus, rose.

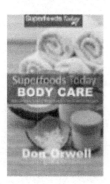

Superfoods Today Cookbook is a Kindle <u>book</u> that contains over 160 Superfoods recipes created with 100% Superfoods ingredients. Most of the meals can be prepared in under 30 minutes and some are really quick ones that can be done in 10 minutes only. Each recipe combines Superfoods ingredients that deliver astonishing amounts of antioxidants, essential fatty acids (like omega-3), minerals, vitamins, and more.

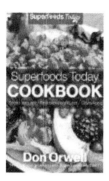

Superfoods Today Smoothies is a Kindle Superfoods Smoothies <u>book</u> with over 70+ 100% Superfoods smoothies. Featured are Red, Purple, Green and Yellow Smoothies

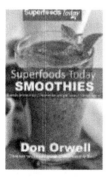

Superfoods Today Salads is a Kindle <u>book</u> that contains over 60 Superfoods Salads recipes created with 100% Superfoods ingredients. Most of the salads can be prepared in 10 minutes and most are measured for two. Each recipe combines Superfoods ingredients that deliver astonishing amounts of antioxidants, essential fatty acids (like omega-3), minerals, vitamins, and more.

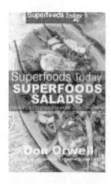

Superfoods Today Kettlebells is a Kindle Kettlebells beginner's <u>book</u> aimed at 30+ office workers who want to improve their health and build stronger body without fat.

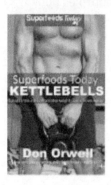

Superfoods Today Red Smoothies is a Kindle Superfoods Smoothies book with more than 40 Red Smoothies.

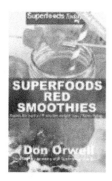

Superfoods Today 14 Days Detox is a Kindle Superfoods Detox book that gives you 2 week Superfoods Detox meal plan and recipes for Detox success.

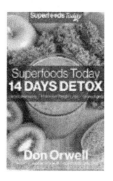

Superfoods Today Yellow Smoothies is a Kindle Superfoods Smoothies book with more than 40 Yellow Smoothies.

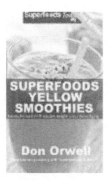

Superfoods Today Green Smoothies is a Kindle Superfoods Smoothies book with more than 35 Green Smoothies.

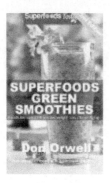

Superfoods Today Purple Smoothies is a Kindle Superfoods Smoothies
book with more than 40 Purple Smoothies.

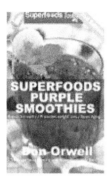

Superfoods Cooking For Two is a Kindle book that contains over 150
Superfoods recipes for two created with 100% Superfoods ingredients.

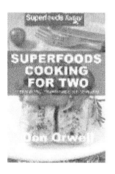

Nighttime Eater is a Kindle <u>book</u> that deals with Nighttime Eating Syndrome (NES). Don Orwell is a life-long Nighttime Eater that has lost his weight with Superfoods and engineered a solution around Nighttime Eating problem. Don still eats at night☺. Don't fight your nature, you can continue to eat at night, be binge free and maintain low weight.

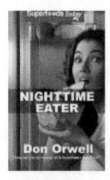

Superfoods Today Smart Carbs 20 Days Detox is a Kindle Superfoods <u>book</u> that will teach you how to detox your body and start losing weight with Smart Carbs. The book has over 470+ pages with over 160+ 100% Superfoods recipes.

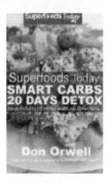

Superfoods Today Vegetarian Salads is a Kindle book that contains over 40 Superfoods Vegetarian Salads recipes created with 100% Superfoods ingredients. Most of the salads can be prepared in 10 minutes and most are measured for two.

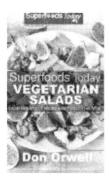

Superfoods Today Vegan Salads is a Kindle book that contains over 30 Superfoods Vegan Salads recipes created with 100% Superfoods ingredients. Most of the salads can be prepared in 10 minutes and most are measured for two.

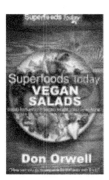

Superfoods Today Soups & Stews is a Kindle book that contains over 70 Superfoods Soups and Stews recipes created with 100% Superfoods ingredients.

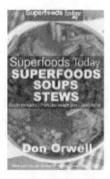

Superfoods Desserts is a Kindle Superfoods Desserts book with more than 60 Superfoods Recipes.

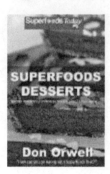

Smoothies for Diabetics is a Kindle <u>book</u> that contains over 70 Superfoods Smoothies adjusted for diabetics.

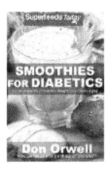

50 Shades of Superfoods for Two is a Kindle <u>book</u> that contains over 150 Superfoods recipes for two created with 100% Superfoods ingredients.

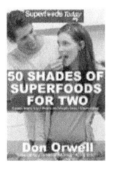

50 Shades of Smoothies is a Kindle <u>book</u> that contains over 70 Superfoods Smoothies.

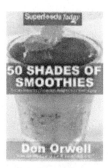

50 Shades of Superfoods Salads is a Kindle <u>book</u> that contains over 60 Superfoods Salads recipes created with 100% Superfoods ingredients. Most of the salads can be prepared in 10 minutes and most are measured for two. Each recipe combines Superfoods ingredients that deliver astonishing amounts of antioxidants, essential fatty acids (like omega-3), minerals, vitamins, and more.

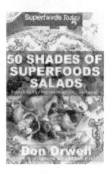

Superfoods Vegan Desserts is a Kindle Vegan Dessert book with 100% Vegan Superfoods Recipes.

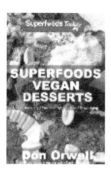

Desserts for Two is a Kindle Superfoods Desserts book with more than 40 Superfoods Desserts Recipes for two.

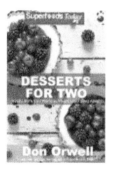

Superfoods Paleo Cookbook is a Kindle Paleo <u>book</u> with more than 150 100% Superfoods Paleo Recipes.

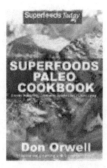

Superfoods Breakfasts is a Kindle Superfoods <u>book</u> with more than 40 100% Superfoods Breakfasts Recipes.

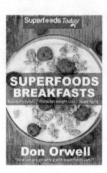

Superfoods Dump Dinners is a Kindle Superfoods <u>book</u> with Superfoods Dump Dinners Recipes.

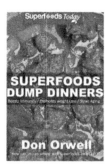

Healthy Desserts is a Kindle Desserts <u>book</u> with more than 50 100% Superfoods Healthy Desserts Recipes.

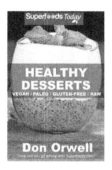

Superfoods Salads in a Jar is a Kindle Salads in a Jar <u>book</u> with more than 35 100% Superfoods Salads Recipes.

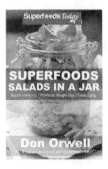

Smoothies for Kids is a Kindle Smoothies <u>book</u> with more than 80 100% Superfoods Smoothies for Kids Recipes.

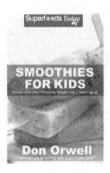

Vegan Cookbook for Beginners is a Kindle Vegan <u>book</u> with more than 75 100% Superfoods Vegan Recipes.

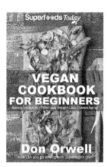

Vegetarian Cooking for Beginners is a Kindle Vegetarian <u>book</u> with more than 150 100% Superfoods Paleo Recipes.

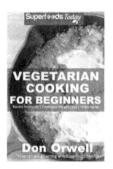

Foods for Diabetics is a Kindle <u>book</u> with more than 170 100% Superfoods Diabetics Recipes.

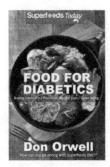

Made in the USA
Las Vegas, NV
22 February 2022

44373424R00246